THE METABOLIC BASIS OF SURGICAL CARE

The Metabolic Basis of Surgical Care

WILLIAM F. WALKER
Ch.M., F.R.C.S.(Ed), F.R.C.S.(Eng)
Consultant Surgeon, Royal Infirmary, Dundee
Hon. Senior Lecturer in Surgery, University of Dundee

IVAN D. A. JOHNSTON
M.Ch., F.R.C.S.(Eng)
Professor of Surgery, University of Newcastle-upon-Tyne
Surgeon, Royal Victoria Infirmary, Newcastle-upon-Tyne

WILLIAM HEINEMANN MEDICAL BOOKS LTD

First Published 1971
© W. F. Walker and I. D. A. Johnston 1971

ISBN 0 433 34580 2

Printed and bound in Great Britain by R. J. Acford Ltd., Industrial Estate, Chichester, Sussex

Contents

Foreword

During the past twenty-five years, since the end of the second world war, there have been surgical advances of the first magnitude, notably in relation to diseases of the heart and blood vessels and in tissue and organ replacement. These new ventures have depended in a large measure on greater understanding of the disturbances which follow severe injury or operation. The ability of the surgical team to maintain the homeostasis of their patients after major operation has been the key to success.

These disturbances are highly complex, involving endocrinological, haemodynamic and nutritional changes whose nature is as yet imperfectly understood though they are the subject of intense research activity in many centres. Each year brings some fragment of new knowledge which sheds a little more light on their nature.

The authors of this monograph are not mere compilers of other men's ideas. Both have made important basic contributions to the subject about which they write and both continue to pursue active research programmes. Their writing, therefore, has the unmistakable stamp of authority and their book will prove a valuable companion for all who have responsibility for the after care of surgical patients.

Professor D. M. Douglas, M.B.E., Ch.M., M.S., F.R.C.S., P.R.C.S.E.
The Royal College of Surgeons, Edinburgh.

There is a circumstance attending accidental injury which does not belong to disease, namely, that the injury done has, in all cases, a tendency to produce both the disposition and means of a cure.

JOHN HUNTER, 1794

Preface

The surgeon's responsibility extends beyond the technical details of operations and includes an understanding of disorders of metabolism which may require correction before surgery is possible, or may follow in the postoperative period. The purpose of this book is to give a concise account of the composition and metabolism of the body in health and disease. An attempt has been made to simplify the presentation without introducing inaccuracy due to over-simplification. Didacticism may on occasions of necessity take the place of a detailed argument about different theories or therapy.

The choice of emphasis was often difficult and many omissions occur. A full account of all the subjects dealt with would have enlarged the book considerably and perhaps confused many readers. We can but state that at the time of writing the statements were acceptable to us and to our colleagues who kindly read and criticised the manuscript.

Good surgical care requires not only a knowledge of the basic composition of the body and the changes in fluid and electrolytes which follow injury or operation but also of the physiology of the circulatory system and the organs involved in metabolism and excretion. We hope that the final section on special problems based, as it is, on physiology and clinical practice will be helpful in the management of critically ill patients.

This book is offered to clinicians who have the responsibility for the day to day care of patients in hospital. Students preparing for their final examination or doing clinical clerkships may find the simple approach to the problem appealing. The junior hospital doctors who face the primary examination in applied basic sciences may find the necessary blend of physiology and clinical medicine useful. Finally, the more senior members of staff may find here and there some suggestions which will help in the care of their ill patients.

We must record our indebtedness to our mentors Professor F. C. Moore (Boston), Professor D. M. Douglas and Professor K. G. Lowe (Dundee), and Professor R. B. Welbourn (London). We are also indebted to our colleagues in Dundee and Newcastle for much helpful criticism of the manuscript and to Mr. Michael Lyall, F.R.C.S. who undertook the arduous job of proof-reading. Most of the illustrations were drawn by Miss Benstead medical artist in the University of Dundee. Others were the work of the Department of Medical Art in the University of Newcastle all of whom we would wish to thank. We cannot forget the help received from the many typists and from Mr. Murray Ettle the Senior Technician in the Department of Surgery, Dundee for his photographic assistance.

1: Body Composition in Health and Disease

It is a sobering thought that the human body is composed merely of water, proteins, fat, carbohydrates and a mixture of elements and salts. Water, the principal component, is present throughout. The organic components are almost entirely intracellular or in the plasma. The inorganic components are both intra and extra cellular, but their concentration in the two compartments is different (Figs. 1 and 2).

This differential is maintained by the cell membranes at the expense of much energy. The mechanics and control of the passage of ions across the cell membrane and the energy expenditure involved is probably one of the most fascinating and little understood mechanisms in the body.

Knowledge of body composition has come to a certain extent from cadaver analysis but mainly from the use of radio-isotopes as tracers. The practical value of such knowledge is variable. Some of it, especially in relation to intravascular volumes, total body water (T.B.W.) and extracellular fluid (E.C.F.) is of considerable interest; other values such as total exchangeable ions have less clinical interest but may provide a basis for our knowledge of the effects of disease and trauma on body physiology and may help in the understanding of more complex metabolic disorders.

Concept of Body Spaces

From the point of view of body composition it is convenient to consider the body as being composed of a number of spaces. This is largely conceptual rather than anatomical as these spaces are defined by areas containing the radio-isotopes at a specific point in time when a dynamic equilibrium exists. Adequate time must be allowed for the equilibration of the isotopes throughout the body spaces.

Principles of Measurement

The most common technique uses radio-isotopes or certain substances which are distributed virtually entirely within the body space concerned. The tracer (isotope or chemical marker) is added to an unknown volume of fluid (tracee) in which it must be mixed adequately. The concentration

1

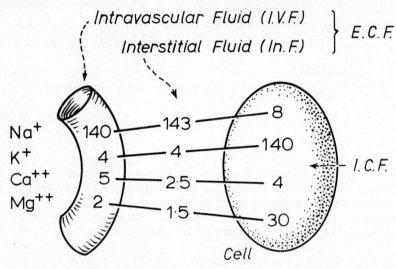

Fig. 1. Cation concentrations in body fluids in mEq/L.

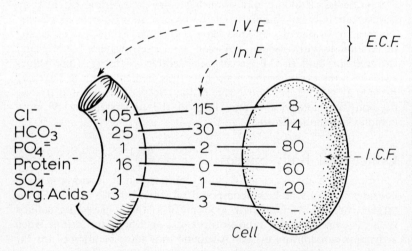

Fig. 2. Anion concentrations in body fluids in mEq/L.

of the tracer in a known quantity of the solution is then estimated and by simple dilution principles the total unknown volume (tracee) can be estimated.

Another technique is by whole body counting which can measure the naturally occurring radioactive isotopes in the body. It needs elaborate and costly apparatus and is therefore of limited value. Its most common use is in measuring total body potassium.

Using the radio-isotopes it is possible to measure not only the body spaces but also the ionic masses. The values of these are shown in Table 1. It must be remembered that these are approximate figures. They may be accepted as "normal" in this context in much the same way as we accept the normal arterial blood pH as being 7·4. For more detailed figures with ranges and correlation data, reference should be made to Moore et al (1963), Moore (1967).

Body Spaces
Total Body Water (T.B.W.)

This is measured by using tritiated water or deuterium oxide as tracers and varies according to the age, sex and total body fat of the patient. In newborn infants it accounts for about 75% of body weight, in adult males about 55% and females 50%. The value for infants falls within the first 2 years. These sex differences are due mainly to the higher fat content in the female since total body water varies inversely with the amount of adipose tissue which is largely anhydrous. Although not strictly correct a figure of 60% of body weight is acceptable for clinical calculations. Water is distributed in the body in two main spaces. The intracellular fluid (I.C.F.) comprises about 40% of the body weight and the extracellular fluid (E.C.F.) accounts for 20%. These figures are somewhat less for I.C.F. and slightly more for E.C.F. Table 1. The E.C.F. is divided further into interstitial fluid (15%) and

Table 1.

Body Fluid Compartments

Component	Volume		Body Weight	
	Male	*Female*	*Male*	*Female*
Total Body Water (T.B.W.)	40L	30L	55%	50%
Intracellular Fluid (I.C.F.)	23L	16L	32%	27%
Extracellular Fluid (E.C.F.)	17L	14L	23%	23%

plasma (5%). The functional importance of these compartments is related inversely to their size. The effect of body fat on total body water is important when estimating fluid replacement.

The water of all non-fat tissue is relatively constant (mean 72%) whereas fat only contains about 20% water by weight. Water may vary then from as little as 40% of body weight in a very obese person to 70% in a lean individual. The fat content has important clinical significance. A 70 Kg man will have 42 litres of water but in an obese person of similar stature and weight the body fat might be 35% of the total weight and the water content would be only 32 litres. Any abnormal loss of water by vomiting or diarrhoea would be less well tolerated in the fat subject. Females respond differently to water loss than males because of the fat ratio differences between the sexes.

Extracellular Fluid (E.C.F.)

The tracers used to measure this space are radiobromine (82 Br), the chemical compound thiocyanate, or a sugar like inulin. As inulin is not metabolised and is excreted rapidly in the urine, a constant infusion technique is required. Other substances such as thiosulphate and sulphate (35 SO_4) have also been used successfully.

The transcellular fluid or third space consists of the cerebrospinal fluid, pleural and peritoneal fluids, secretions of alimentary glands, and intestinal contents. This further division of the E.C.F. is small (less than 3% of body weight), but capable in certain circumstances of increasing remarkably to reduce the effective E.C.F. It is not possible to measure this space accurately, although it may be important in conditions such as intestinal obstruction or paralytic ileus.

Blood Volume

The red cell volume and plasma volume may be measured separately or as is more usual the plasma volume is measured and allowance made for the haematocrit.

Table 2.

Intravascular Volumes

Component	Body Weight	
Total Blood Volume	70 ml/Kg	7%
Red Cell Volume	25 ml/kg	2%
Plasma Volume	45 ml/kg	5%

Red Cell Volume:— Red cells removed from the patient are labelled with radio-phosphorus (^{32}P) or radiochromium (^{51}Cr). They are washed, resuspended in saline and reinjected into the patient. After ten minutes equilibration a further sample of blood is removed and its activity measured. From these measurements the dilution may be assessed and the total red cell mass obtained. This is approximately 2–4% of body weight.

Plasma Volume:— Two substances are commonly used to measure this—Evans Blue (T–1824) and radio-iodinated serum albumin (R.I.S.A.). Both of these tag the circulating plasma protein. The plasma volume is approximately 5% of the body weight. In clinical practice rapid and serial estimates can now be done using purpose built instruments such as the volemetron which have a built-in mechanism for correcting for background counts.

The value of blood volume and plasma volume measurements is so well known that it hardly needs emphasis here. Along with measurement of central venous pressure (right atrial pressure) they constitute the most significant advances in the study of shock. Various methods have been described for measurement of these simultaneously with the E.C.F. volume (Moore et al, 1963 and Hoye, 1967).

Body Ionic Masses

Sodium

Measurement of total body sodium by isotopes is not possible, because almost one third is in the skeleton and not readily exchangeable. The remaining sodium, the exchangeable and thus dynamically active sodium, is measured by tracer techniques using radioactive sodium (^{24}Na). Normally, it amounts to 2800 mEq or 40 mEq/Kg. Of this, about 1500 mEq (140 mEq/1) is in the E.C.F. and about 1300 mEq (8 mEq/1) in the I.C.F.

Potassium

The total body potassium and the total exchangeable potassium (Ke), unlike sodium, are almost identical and amount to approximately 3200 mEq in an adult man (48 mEq/Kg). They are a little less in the female (40 mEq/Kg) because she has a higher content of fat in the body and consequently a lower level of potassium containing lean tissue. The extracellular space contains about 60 mEq of K at a concentration of 4·5 mEq/1. The intracellular K concentration is about 140 mEq/1. At present the measurements of body K are made using a short life istotope ^{42}K.

Magnesium

This is the other main intracellular cation which is of considerable importance in enzyme activity. The total body magnesium, from cadaver analysis, is estimated at 2,000 mEq in a 70 Kg man. Much of this magnesium is in the bone. The normal serum concentration is 1·5–1·8 mEq/1. The magnesium concentration in the cells is much higher and is about 30 mEq/1.

Calcium

Estimations of total body calcium have proved difficult. The results of cadaver analysis has varied widely under differing circumstances. Radio-isotope studies were hampered by the long life of ^{45}Ca but have proved more possible using ^{47}Ca which has a short half-life (4·7 days) or ^{85}S which behaves as a tracer for calcium. In the adult, there is about 1000 g of calcium (1·6% of body weight). This is mainly in the skeleton. The calcium content is only 0·8% of body weight at birth, rising especially at puberty and in adolescence. The extracellular calcium concentration is 5 mEq/l; intracellular calcium is 4 mEq/l.

Derived Data

As already described, total body water, extracellular water, total body sodium and potassium can be measured using the appropriate isotope. From these and the total body weight further calculations of the body composition can be made by accepting a few assumptions. Thus one can derive fat-free body (F.F.B.), total body solids (T.B.S.) fat free solids (F.F.S.) etc. As these are of little clinical value, they will not be considered here. Reference should be made to Moore et al, 1963.

Control of Body Composition

The composition of the body is not static but varies with body development and as a result of stress in the form of disease and trauma.

Normal development from birth consists of a gradual diminution in the T.B.W. as a percentage of the body weight reaching its lowest in old age. The I.C.F. space increases as a percentage of body weight with the development of body cells especially muscle cells and reaches its highest in the muscular male adult and then diminishes with age. Apart from these normal variations other changes occur as a result of starvation, obesity, disease or trauma and are discussed below.

Before considering them it is pertinent to look at the factors governing control of water and electrolytes as these also control the body spaces.

Control of Body Water

When water is taken by mouth it is absorbed rapidly passing into the blood stream. From there it is excreted just as rapidly by the kidney. If large amounts of water are drunk a diuresis ensues. But, if the intake is too large and too rapid (especially if given intravenously) for the kidneys to deal with it, the water passes through the basement membrane of the capillaries into the E.C.F. and possibly into the I.C.F. through the cell membrane. These membranes are semi-permeable in that water is freely diffusible through them, electrolytes less so, and plasma proteins almost not at all. The cell membrane is semi-permeable to water but passage of ions across it requires more than simple diffusion. Ionic pumps are involved, such as the Sodium pump, which require energy for their action as mentioned already.

The movement of water also occurs in the opposite direction, i.e. from the cell to E.C.F. and plasma, so that a dynamic equilibrium exists between the various body compartments in the steady state.

The factors operating in the control of body water are thus:—

1. Factors controlling absorption from the gut, e.g. availability of water, size of intestinal lumen (distension diminishes absorption), state of epithelium and rate of movement through the intestine.
2. Ability of the kidneys to excrete water.
3. Osmolality.
   This is the main factor controlling the shift of fluids and electrolytes between compartments.
4. Insensible losses by respiration and through the skin and faeces.

Absorption Factors

Intensive interest has been shown recently in the ability of the intestine to absorb water and electrolytes. This interest is not new but has been stimulated by the use of radioisotopes in absorption studies, and the opportunity presented, in surgical patients especially, to study the passage of these isotopes to and fro across the bowel wall. Under various conditions we are normally little aware that about 8 litres (almost 3 times the plasma volume) of alimentary secretions are passed daily into the intestinal tract and reabsorbed. Little aware, that is, until the reabsorptive capacity is interfered with or reduced by dilatation of the bowel as in intestinal obstruction or paralytic ileus. Then the loss of fluid into the dilated gut reduces the plasma volume rapidly and may produce shock.

Absorption of water and electrolytes mainly from the small bowel is not a passive phenomenon, but is influenced by mineralo-corticoid activity (Fordtran, 1966, Parson, 1967, Shields, 1968).

Much has yet to be learned about the effect of different pathological conditions on the absorptive capacity of the gut.

Renal Regulation of Water

Water passing through the glomerulus into the proximal tubule is largely absorbed there with sodium. As the remainder passes down the descending limb of Henle's loop some of it diffuses passively into the interstitium. In the ascending limb no water passes out as the membrane there is impermeable. Sodium is pumped out into the interstitium raising the osmolality and by providing a hyperosmolar medium allows the loop to act as a countercurrent multiplier system. In the distal convoluted tubule water is absorbed with sodium in response to Aldosterone. Finally as it passes into the collecting ducts more of the water passes out into the interstitium under the action of anti-diuretic hormone (A.D.H.) which encourages the production of a hyperosmolar urine.

Osmolality

The main factor controlling shifts of fluids and electrolytes between body compartments is the osmolality of the spaces, which are all iso-osmolar. When the osmolarity rises in one compartment due to the increase in solute or diminution of water, then water will pass in from the other compartments to restore iso-osmolality. These two terms are confused frequently: osmolarity represents the solute concentration per litre of solution whereas osmolality refers to the solute concentration per unit of total weight of solvent. As the difference between the two is very small in the body fluids, they can be regarded as interchangeable. Osmolality is dependent on the number and size of molecules present in the solution. As the electrolytes have small molecules they are mainly responsible for the osmolality of the body compartments. Sodium, the principal ion in the E.C.F., is mainly responsible for its osmolality whereas K is responsible for cellular osmolality.

The plasma osmolality is 280–310 mos/1 (2 × Na$^+$ concentration). Apart from sodium and potassium the other crystalloids which are present throughout the E.C.F. and I.C.F. make up the total osmolality of these spaces. This is especially so with regard to sugar and urea and an allowance for these can be made in the following formula:

$$\text{Posm.} = (\text{Na} + \text{K}) \times 2 + \left(\frac{\text{Urea}}{6} + \frac{\text{CHO}}{18} \right) \text{ where 6 and 18 convert}$$

the concentration of urea and CHO from mg per cent to mEq/1. The plasma has the added effect of the plasma proteins the molecules of which however, because of their large size have a small osmotic effect (6–12 mosmol/l). Even so, this is important as they are present only in the intravascular component. The osmotic or oncotic pressure of plasma and the hydrostatic pressure in the capillaries largely govern the interchange of fluid between the circulation and the interstitial fluid. This is covered by Starling's law which states that the balance between hydrostatic pressure, colloid osmotic pressure, and osmotic pressure of the interstitial fluid at the arterial and venular end of the capillary controls the extent and rate of flow.

Sodium regulates the shift of fluid between the interstitial fluid and the cell.

Body Composition in Abnormal States

1. Starvation and Wasting Disease

In starvation associated for example with carcinoma of the oesophagus a process of cannibalism occurs where fat and protein is broken down slowly to provide energy for normal body metabolism. This leads to a decrease in intracellular water (as the cells decrease) and an increase in the extracellular water which ultimately may become so excessive as to be apparent clinically as starvation oedema. Nitrogen will be excreted in the urine, and, as there is virtually no intake, this represents the wasting of cells in the lean tissues. Negative nitrogen balance is accompanied also by negative K balance and diminution in total exchangeable K. The excess of water comes mainly from the oxidation of the fat as well as from lysis of the lean tissue.

The kidney inappropriately restricts its excretion of salt and water, making the waterlogging process worse.

2. Acute Illness and Trauma

The same process takes place here but in a much more rapid way especially if the trauma or illness is associated with sepsis. Large negative nitrogen balances of 20 g/day may occur and as each g of nitrogen represents roughly 6 g of protein this is a loss of 120 g/protein/ day or approximately 1 Kg of wet lean tissue. Fat oxidation will also be increased so that water can rapidly accumulate. This with a low urine output is responsible for the dilution hyponatraemia seen post-operatively. Additional water given intravenously must be administered with caution and should contain some salt. Severe illness and trauma will thus be associated with diminution of fat content of the body, and in exchangeable K. The E.C.F. will be increased until the diuresis takes place.

3. Third Space Effect

This term is given to these cases in which there is accumulation of fluid outside the normal recognised body spaces. This loss of fluid is most important clinically. A classic example of this is in burns when "burns oedema" may be present, and fluid accumulates in the sub-cutaneous tissues presumably due to damage to the capillaries by heat. The body weight following burns actually increases initially instead of falling as might be expected. Fluid also accumulates in the limbs following deep vein thrombosis; in the gut in paralytic ileus or obstruction; in the abdominal cavity in ascites. The third space expands at the expense of the plasma volume which is reduced and shock may be evident.

4. Haemorrhage

Loss of whole blood reduces the intravascular component of the E.C.F. space. Immediately the repair process begins in the capillaries, where water is brought in from the interstitial space to make up for the volume lost. This process takes 24–48 hours to be complete depending on the amounts involved. The red cell volume is diminished in respect of the plasma volume which is increased by the transcapillary filling. Replacement of red cells, a more gradual process, restores the situation to normal.

5. Heart Disease

The basic compositional changes in heart disease are a reflection of decreased water and salt excretion and tissue anoxia. The amount of change is dependent naturally on the degree to which these two factors are affected. Thus in cardiac disease with little haemodynamic change, as in congenital cardiac septal defects, there may be little or no change. At the other extreme in long standing chronic cardiac failure with valve destruction, the changes are considerable.

Retention of water is greater than that of salt. Both lead to expansion of E.C.F. with a fall in ratio of I.C.W. and T.B.W. and a rise in exchangeable sodium. Some of the water will come from oxidation of fat where a low calorie intake is present. Excess water produces haemodilution and hypotonicity and, despite an increase in exchangeable sodium, reduces the plasma sodium. The plasma volume is increased.

The poor circulation in cardiac failure produces some degree of tissue anoxia. Tissue breakdown occurs with excretion of nitrogen and potassium. The body cell mass decreases especially in the more chronic states with therefore a fall in exchangeable potassium (Ke) and a fall in the ratio of Ke to T.B.W. and to body weight. Despite this, the plasma K may be normal or even slightly raised.

Where pulmonary disease is present, and in cyanotic heart disease such as Fallot's Tetralogy the red cell volume increases. This further augments the increased blood volume. Severe lung disease will lead to chronic respiratory acidosis with risk of a further rise in plasma K.

Operation in a patient with abnormal body composition can be dangerous. Further retention of salt and water will follow and hyperkalaemia may be produced in the early post-operative phase. Digitalis and diuretics help to return the E.C.F. and plasma volume to normal. But unless K supplementation is given there may be a further reduction in Ke with risk of hypokalaemia. Changes in plasma K following operation can only be detected by careful repeated measurements.

6. Hepatic Failure

This produces changes in body composition almost identical with those of chronic cardiac failure and are due also to excessive water retention, above that of sodium. Again an inappropriate A.D.H. effect on the kidney is postulated. This and tissue wasting leads to loss of body fat, loss of lean body mass and increased E.C.F. In advanced liver failure there is a severe degree of hypotonicity with a dramatic fall in plasma sodium. A sodium level of less than 125 mEq/1 is regarded as ominous (Hecker and Sherlock, 1965).

7. Renal Failure

The compositional picture in acute renal failure is related to the inability to get rid of water whether endogenously produced or given by mouth or intravenously. Excess fluids will increase the hypotonicity of body fluids. There is a rise in E.C.F. and exchangeable Na. The Ke is normal but the plasma K may rise especially if metabolic acidosis is present. In chronic renal failure the risk of over-hydration and over-salting is greater than in acute failure. Unless there is marked restriction in fluid and electrolyte intake the E.C.F. will rise and the I.C.F. will fall. Usually the change in I.C.F. is small as malnutrition is uncommon and the lean body mass is not eroded. The plasma changes are a fall in red cell volume and in the sodium level and a rise in plasma K. The K change of course is accentuated by metabolic acidosis and with this the calcium level may fall and phosphate rise in time to produce secondary hyperparathyroidism.

8. *Effect of Hot Climate*

The problem presented by a hot climate is one of loss of water and salt by sweating. As acclimatisation occurs it takes a higher temperature to produce sweating and the loss of salt is less.

When Europeans move to tropical conditions there is an increase in T.B.W. and in the daily turnover of water. The T.B.W. rose from 43·5 to 47·0 litres in one study despite a fall in total body weight of 2 Kg (McFarlane, 1964). This was accompanied by increased daily turnover of water from 3·7L/day, to nearly 7·0L/day, and the E.C.F. increased by 20%. In children who have a greater body surface area the rise in T.B.W. and water turnover is more marked.

Increased external heat produces vasodilatation of skin vessels with loss of heat by radiation and when sweating occurs by evaporation. The loss of salt and water in the sweat is compensated for initially by a shift in fluid from E.C.F. to plasma. But, if sweating proceeds the plasma volume will fall. As more water than salt is lost the plasma becomes hypertonic and thirst is experienced. The osmoreceptors are stimulated and A.D.H. is liberated to produce oliguria (McFarlane and Robertson, 1957).

The normal salt loss from the body surface in the unacclimatised is 90 mEq/l of sweat; in the acclimatised this drops to nearly 10 mEq/l.

The importance of these observations in surgery was evaluated by Tinckler, 1966, who studied the problem in the Persian Gulf at temperatures of 90–95°F. He found that following operation the acclimatised patient required about 2 to 4 litres of 5% Dextrose daily to make up losses from skin and lungs. Saline was required in the unacclimatised patient and for each litre of fluid given an extra 250 ml of normal saline was required to make up for the loss of salt in the sweat.

REFERENCES

Moore, F. D., Olesen, K. H., McMurray, J. D., Parker, H. V., Ball, M. R. and Boyden, C. M. (1963). The Body Cell Mass and its supporting environment. Philadelphia: Saunders.

Moore, F. D. (1967). Body Composition and its measurement in vivo. *Brit. J. Surg.*, **54**, 431.

Hoye, R. C. (1967). Simultaneous measurements of red cells, plasma and extracellular fluid volume in the surgical patient. *J. Lab. & Clin. Med.*, **69**, 683.

Fordtran, J. S. and Dietschy, J. M. (1966). Water and electrolyte movement in the intestine. *Gastroenterology*, **50**, 263.

Parsons, D. S. (1967). Salt and Water absorption by the intestinal tract. *Brit. Med. Bull.*, **23**, 252.

Shields, R. (1968). Syndrome of water and electrolyte depletion of intestinal origins. *Scot. Med. J.*, **13**, 122.

Hecker, R. and Sherlock, S. (1956). Electrolyte and circulatory changes in terminal liver failure. *Lancet*, **2**, 1121.

McFarlane, W. V. (1964). Environmental physiology and psychology in arid conditions. *Proc. of Lucknow Conf. U.N.B.S.C.O. Paris*, 43.

McFarlane, W. V. and Robinson, K. W. N. (1957). Seasonal changes in plasma antidiuretic activity produced by standard heat stimulus. *J. Physiol.*, **135**, 1.

Tinckler, L. F. (1966). Fluid and electrolyte observations in tropical surgical practice. *Brit. Med. J.*, **1**, 1263.

2: Water and Electrolyte Metabolism

The previous chapter has dealt with the composition of the body in respect of water and electrolytes and the effects of disease on this. Here, we are concerned with the physiological activity of water and electrolytes, the mechanism controlling their presence and distribution, and finally, the abnormal patterns due to trauma or disease.

Water is the universal solvent in which is dissolved the electrolytes in varying concentrations throughout the body compartments. The cell membrane acts as the differential which maintains the electrolyte concentrations within and without the cell. These concentrations, by their osmotic activity, control the passage of water.

Water

There are two main ways of expressing the daily intake of water, either in terms of surface area as 800 ml/m²/day, or body weight as ml/Kg. The most sensible way is in relation to surface area, as water is lost from the skin by evaporation. This, however, requires the use of tables for calculations and although more exact, is largely superseded in clinical practice by the more easily measured weight of the patient.

In babies, who have a much greater relative surface area, an intake of 100 ml/Kg is required. As the child grows the amount diminishes to about 80 ml/Kg at 1–2 years: 60 ml/Kg at 2–5 years until over 5 years, when the same figure is used as for adults, i.e. 40 ml/Kg. The fluid intake normally comes from three sources (Table 3): oral liquids (1200 ml/day); water derived from solid food (1000 ml/day); and water of oxidation of food and body tissues (300 ml/day). This approximate total intake in the adult is balanced by the following daily losses: urine (1400 ml/day), from lungs and skin (1000 ml/day), and in the faeces (100 ml/day). A wide range of intake and output exists under normal conditions and in abnormal conditions, such as tracheostomy with hyperpnoea, hyperpyrexia, vomiting, ileus or diarrhoea, the losses by the various routes may be markedly increased. When this happens, the urine output is adjusted to maintain, if possible, daily fluid balance. The two components are obligatory water required for the excretion of solutes and excess or free water which varies with the intake.

The basic data for water is shown in Table 4.

Table 3.

Daily Gains and Losses of Water

Gains	Drink	1,200 ml
	In food	1,000 ml
	From oxidation	300 ml
	Grand Total	2,500 ml
Losses "Unavoidable"		
	Expired Air	400 ml ⎤
	Faeces	100 ml ⎬ Extrarenal Losses
	Skin (insensible)	300 ml ⎦
	Urine (obligatory)	500 ml
	Total	1,300 ml
"Avoidable"	Urine (free)	1,200 ml
	Grand Total	2,500 ml

Table 4.

Basic Data on Water

Body Composition	T.B.W.	I.C.F.	E.C.F.	(I.F. Plasma)
Infant	75% B.W.	45%	30%	(26% 4%)
Adult male	55%	32%	23%	(18% 5%)
Adult female	50%	27%	23%	(18% 5%)
Water Intake				
Infants	60–100 ml/Kg			
Children 5 yrs.	60–80 ml/Kg			
Adults	40 ml/Kg			

N.B. In clinical cases when calculating volumes of fluids to infuse, it is usual to consider the distribution of water in adults in round (if inaccurate) figures

$$viz. \text{ T.B.W.} = 60\% \text{ of body weight in Kg}$$
$$\text{I.C.F.} = 40\% \text{ of body weight in Kg}$$
$$\text{E.C.F.} = 20\% \text{ of body weight in Kg}$$

Effect of Trauma

In abnormal conditions, the daily fluid requirements may have to go up when the losses increase. Following injury, the opposite happens as antidiuretic hormone (A.D.H.) is released as part of the metabolic response to trauma. This produces a fall in urine output with, therefore, retention of water and drops the fluid intake required to 1500–2000 ml/day. If, however, trauma results in an increased extra-renal loss of fluid, as for example, in the development of an ileus or intestinal fistula, then the intake must be adjusted accordingly. It is simply a matter of balancing intake with output. The problem is to estimate the losses with reasonable accuracy.

Control of Water Metabolism

When water is taken by mouth it is absorbed from all parts of the intestinal tract, notably the colon. The water intake is controlled by the thirst mechanism. This is activated when the water content of the body falls without an associated fall in electrolyte, i.e. a state of hypertonicity exists. This could also occur where excess sodium was given in relation to water by the intravenous infusion of hypertonic saline. It is still not completely clear exactly how the mechanism of thirst works but, it is reasonable to suppose that a change in plasma osmolality stimulates an osmo-receptor area in the brain adapted as a "thirst-centre". The same change in osmolality stimulates osmo-receptors in the internal carotid artery so that Anti-Diuretic Hormone is formed in the supra-optic and para-ventricular nuclei of the hypothalamus and is released from the posterior pituitary (Fig. 3). The main effect of A.D.H. is to increase water reabsorption in the distal convoluted tubule and collecting ducts. Increased osmolality is not the only stimulant to A.D.H. release. A decrease in blood volume or in E.C.F. also brings about the release of A.D.H., as does pain, fear, and drugs such as morphine, adrenaline and barbiturate to name a few. The factors affecting A.D.H. and its activity have been reviewed by Zimmerman (1965) and Wakim (1967). The action of pain, fear and drugs, all part of the surgical experience, has particular relevance to the post-operative state when A.D.H. release has been activated and continued by the above. If the patient is on intravenous infusions, he may be overloaded and be less able to deal with this by inhibition of A.D.H. and renal excretion. It has long been recognised that our defence against dehydration is more efficient than against the less common event, water overloading. This is at no time more true than after operation.

Although changes in osmolar constancy are the main forces affecting water metabolism, it should be remembered that water is absorbed and released with the electrolytes, and is necessary for the excretion of solute loads. The prevalent use of Dextrans, Mannitol and diuretics in patients following, or being prepared for, surgery, can all upset the balance of water in the body.

Clinical Water Syndromes

The two abnormal syndromes associated with water metabolism are water depletion (dehydration) and water excess (water intoxication). While these conditions, like the other syndromes in fluid and electrolytes metabolism are described, more or less, as pure syndromes, it is rare

A D H RELEASE

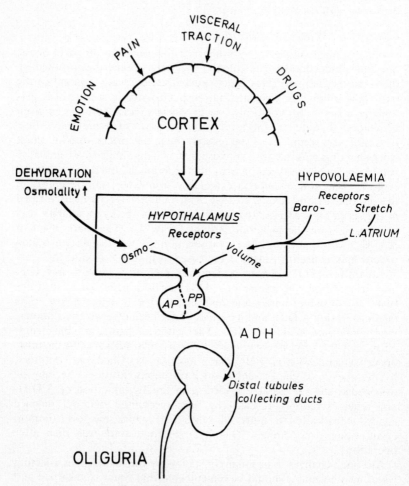

FIG. 3. Mechanism of A.D.H. release.

to find them as such. They are usually part of complex metabolic disorders in which they are merely the principal offender.

I. Water Depletion—Dehydration

In its strictest sense, dehydration means lack of water, and this is the sense used here. All too often in the past, and even now, it is used to describe lack of water and electrolytes. When the water content of the body falls without an associated fall in electrolytes, thirst is experienced due to the hyperosmolar state. Thirst usually means a deficiency of at least 1·5 litres. The urine output falls and as there is still a solute load, the specific gravity and urea concentration rises. The body weight will fall and as starvation is often associated with loss of water over a prolonged period, the weight loss will be greater than that due to water alone. When the water loss is in excess of 4 litres the blood volume diminishes, the pulse speeds up and the blood pressure falls. The withdrawal of water from the tissues to maintain the blood volume initially, results in loss of tissue turgor, loss of elasticity of the skin, and fall in intra-ocular pressure. Cerebral dehydration produces mental confusion and coma from which the patient may not recover.

The effect of loss of water falls predominantly on the I.C.F. rather than the E.C.F. When the blood volume falls, Aldosterone release is stimulated. This causes retention of salt and water which remains in the E.C.F., so sustaining the plasma volume for a time at least.

Changes in blood chemistry are late in pure dehydration and, if present, mean a significant loss of water. The plasma sodium may rise and to a less extent, so also may the haematocrit. The changes in the haematocrit are much less marked than in a salt loss state. In time the blood urea and plasma proteins may increase.

The clinical picture of the patient is one of shrivelling up due to loss of intracellular water. The dry lax skin may be accompanied by a dry mouth, muscle weakness, pulse of weak volume and low blood pressure (a late event). The main problem is to differentiate the skin changes from age and recent loss of weight. This is not always easy as they may be present in addition to dehydration. Thirst is an excellent differential point.

Causes of Water Depletion

There are two broad groups of causes:—diminished intake of water and increased loss.

1. *Diminished intake.* In temperate climates, this is usually the result of inability to swallow as in carcinoma of the oesophagus or in mental or neurological conditions. In hot countries circumstances may arise, as in deserts, where water is just not available.

2. *Increased loss.* The routes of loss are:—

a) *Urine:* Excess water loss in the urine may be seen in diabetes insipidis, chronic nephritis where urine with a very low specific gravity is excreted, and with diuretics where the electrolytes may be replaced intravenously but the water loss is allowed to get out of control.

b) *Skin and lungs:* Hyperventilation from any cause will increase water loss especially if the patient is on a ventilator with a tracheostomy tube in place. To compensate for this ventilators should be humidified and it is possible with humidification to actually gain as much as a litre of water in 24 hours. Sweating due to hyperpyrexia or a hot climate produces a loss of hypotonic sweat.

c) *Faeces:* In severe diarrhoea water loss may predominate although usually the electrolytes, especially potassium, are affected. A loss of water into the gut can also occur when excessively hypertonic diets are given by tube feeding.

Diagnosis

This may be obvious, depending on the cause. Often however, in hospitals in this country, difficulty may be experienced as already mentioned. This is especially so in the confused elderly patients or in patients following surgery.

The three points of greatest value in the differential diagnosis are (1) Thirst—in the conscious patient; (2) low urine volume below 700 ml/day: the differential diagnosis of oliguria is shown in Table 29. (3) A high plasma sodium in the absence of administration of hypertonic saline.

Treatment

Water should be given by mouth or as 5% Dextrose intravenously until thirst disappears, urine volume is increased, and the plasma sodium returns to normal. The rate of administration depends on the condition of the patient. In the elderly or after trauma, there may be some concomitant impairment of renal function, so it is important not to overtreat and swing from dehydration to water intoxication.

As already mentioned, dehydrated patients may also be suffering from starvation and as water is replaced, the question of calories should be entertained. Once the acute water shortage has been treated, intravenous fat and amino acids may be required. This is discussed more fully in Chapter 3.

II. Water Excess—Intoxication

This is the direct opposite of water depletion and, in this condition the body water is increased without an increase in the electrolyte content.

Normally, water intoxication is prevented by an increase in urine volume. It is thus rarely seen without some degree of renal impairment. The use of intravenous solutions create circumstances where water intoxication may occur. A particular example is when gastric suction is used with the replacement of the electrolyte rich fluid by intravenous 5% Dextrose. This produces a hypotonicity of the E.C.F. so that water then shifts into the cells causing them to swell. This particularly affects the cerebral cells and, as a result, curious mental changes may occur. The symptoms vary with the degree and rapidity of the process.

When the accumulation of water is rapid, cerebral symptoms predominate. With a more gradual onset, a vague feeling of weakness is accompanied by lethargy and apathy. The acutely confused patient may be suspected to be suffering from a psychological disturbance or even a small stroke. Convulsions may occur.

An increase in body water leads to an increase in body weight—an unsual and dangerous sign in a surgical patient. The face may appear puffy and slight pitting oedema of the legs may be seen. The circulatory status is unimpaired, indeed there may be a slight increase in blood pressure.

The blood changes are a fall in the haematocrit and also in the plasma sodium which may be less than 120 mEq/L.

Causes of Water Intoxication

1. Overtreatment of dehydration.
2. Excessive I.V. fluids in presence of renal failure.
3. Water replacement of a fluid and electrolyte loss, e.g. gastric aspiration.
4. Excess water in the post-operative period especially after cardiac surgery.

Diagnosis

It should be suspected clinically when neurological signs and symptoms appear unexpectedly, especially in a patient receiving intravenous 5% Dextrose. The presence of a low plasma sodium in a patient with a normal blood pressure, who is obviously not suffering from salt depletion, should alert the clinician. When a patient has cerebral symptoms, a low plasma sodium, and a normal circulation and blood pressure, the diagnosis is practically certain.

Treatment

The acute case requires 100 ml of 5% Saline hourly until the convulsions stop. Repeated plasma sodium estimations should be done to prevent overtreatment, and once it is over 130 mEq/L the hypertonic saline should be stopped and the condition allowed to adjust itself by the renal excretion of water. This can be aided by the use of diuretics.

Isotonic saline is ineffective as it will not correct the hypotonicity of the body fluids. Indeed, its use may be dangerous in this condition.

Electrolytes

Electrolytes are substances which when placed in water, dissociate into ions. These ions have a positive or negative charge according to their attraction to a specific pole of an electrical circuit. Those with a negative charge are attracted to the positive pole and are thus designated anode positive ions (ANIONS). Those with a positive charge are attracted to the cathode negative tube and are called CATIONS.

The ions are distributed throughout the body compartments in a variable fashion as mentioned in Chapter 1. Their distribution is governed to some extent by the distribution of body water, but more especially by the selectivity of the cell membranes. Thus sodium is the main extracellular ion and potassium the main intracellular one (Fig. 1.) The concentration of these ions in the various body spaces produces an osmotic effect which is important in the control of water distribution. Thus water and ions are interdependent.

In clinical practice we are more concerned with the concentration of the ions in the plasma than in the body compartments. This is because measurement of plasma ions is easy whereas their concentration in body compartments requires rather complex procedures. In the plasma the sum of the cations always equals that of the anions. The unit of measurement of the ions—the milliequivalent (mEq/L) measures the chemical combining power of the ion related to the chemical combining capacity of approximately one gram of hydrogen. Thus one mEq of any of the cations is able to react completely with one mEq of any anion. A further term used in discussing electrolyte activity is the milliosmol. This has regard to the osmotic activity of the ions in a

H_2CO3	1.2 mMoL/L
Na^+ 142 mEq.	Cl^- 105 mEq.
	HCO_3^- 24 mEq.
	Pr. 16 mEq.
K^+ 5 mEq.	Org. Acid$^-$ 6 mEq.
Ca^{++} 5 mEq.	$SO_4^=$ 1 mEq.
Mg^{++} 2 mEq.	$PO_4^=$ 2 mEq.

FIG. 4. Ions in the plasma.

solution rather than their chemical combining activity. As mentioned in Chapter 1, the OSMOLARITY of a solution relates the concentrations of the solute per unit of total volume of a solution, i.e. mols/l of solution. In osmolality the concentration of the solute is related to the total weight of the solvent (mols/Kg). For practical purposes in body fluids the two are interchangeable although osmolarity is said to be temperature dependent whereas osmolality is not. The relationship of mOsm to mEq is governed by valency. In the monovalent ions e.g. Na^+, K^+, HCO_3^-, CL^-, P_2^-, Org. Acid$^-$. One mEq. is equal to one mosmol. As regards the BIVALENT ions, Ca^{++}, Mg^{++}, $HPO_4^=$ and $SO_4^=$ 2 mEq equal 1 mosmol.

The concentration of the ions in the plasma is usually represented in columns after the manner of GAMBLE—Fig. 4. The balanced relationship of the Cations and Anions will be emphasised repeatedly in discussion on the ions themselves.

Cations

Sodium

As sodium is the main extracellular cation, its importance in the body economy cannot be overemphasised. Indeed, this is underlined by the careful way in which the body controls sodium metabolism. The main function of sodium is the control and distribution of water throughout the body by its effect on the osmolality of the tissue fluid, which osmolality is dependent on the number of molecules of sodium per unit of water. If sodium is lost, so also is water to maintain osmolality, and if sodium is retained in the body, so also is water to dilute it. It is, of course, possible by infusion of fluids, to upset this normal balance and produce excess of water in the body over that of sodium (water intoxication) and vice versa—hypernatraemia. The basic data on sodium is shown in Table 5.

Control of Body Sodium

This is accomplished by the kidney which is the only practical excretory organ for sodium, and only very small amounts are lost in the sweat or in the stool under normal circumstances. Even so, only about 2% of the filtered sodium is actually passed out in the urine. The rest is reabsorbed by the renal tubules.

Proximal Tubular Absorption:— This is the main site of absorption of sodium where approximately 80% is absorbed. Despite this, our knowledge of the mechanisms involved is limited. Certain factors are important and two of these are the hydrostatic pressure and plasma protein osmotic pressure in the peri-tubular venous capillaries. A further factor is the change in the volume of the E.C.F. which affects reabsorption markedly. Apart from these, there is much evidence to support the concept of an unknown hormone, released by changes in E.C.F. volume, on the proximal tubule (De Wardener et al, 1961). This salt retaining hormone differs from any of the present known hormones acting on the kidney and the evidence for its existence has been admirably reviewed recently by De Wardener (1969).

Table 5.

Basic Data on Sodium

Composition Body

Total body sodium	— 4000 mEq
Exchangeable sodium (Nae)	— 2800 mEq or 40 mEq/Kg
Intracellular (3%)	— 250 mEq or 3·5 mEq/Kg
Extracellular (57%)	— 1600 mEq or 23 mEq/Kg
Bone sodium (40%)	— 900 mEq or 130 mEq/Kg

Balance—Daily

Sodium intake	— 100 mEq/day or 6·0g NaCl
Sodium ouput	— 80 mEq/day—Urine
	10 mEq/day—Faeces
	10 mEq/day—Sweat

Concentration in:—

Body Fluids—Plasma	138–142 mEq/L	
Cell	8 mEq/L	
C.S.F.	130 mEq/L	

Intestinal Juices

Saliva	10 mEq/L
Gastric juice	60 mEq/L
Bile	150 mEq/L
Pancreatic juice	140 mEq/L
Small bowel	120 mEq/L

Distal Tubular Absorption:— This is the "fine" adjustment mechanism responsible for about 20% of sodium reabsorption. The Aldosterone responsible for this is released by the RENIN-ANGIOTENSIN system (Fig. 5). In this, the renal afferent arterioles and juxtaglomerular apparatus respond to changes in renal arterial pressure, and/or renal blood flow, and possibly to intracellular sodium concentration, by releasing RENIN which acts on a plasma substrate to produce the octapeptide ANGIOTENSIN II. This stimulates the release of Aldosterone from the adrenal cortex. Aldosterone increases the reabsorption of sodium in the distal tubule and increases the secretion of potassium and hydrogen ion from that site. This is not a sodium for potassium exchange as the potassium excretion may persist after sodium excretion has returned to normal.

Effects of Trauma

The retention of sodium after injury usually begins immediately, reaches its maximum by the second day and lasts for 4–6 days or even longer, depending on the age of the patient, the severity of trauma, and the presence of complications. This response is one of the most constant features of the metabolic response to trauma and is mediated through the release of Aldosterone. While the response is constant, it can be altered and nearly eliminated by maintaining the E.C.F. volume and arterial and venous pressures as near normal as possible. Indeed, the greater the care exercised in controlling the body's homeostatic mechanism, the less will this response be evident (Walker, 1967).

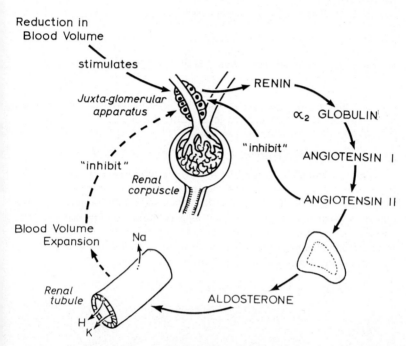

FIG. 5. Renin angiotensin system.

Retention of sodium is accompanied by retention of water. This is often in excess of that of sodium retention, so that the excess water can produce a small fall in plasma sodium to levels about 130 mEq/L. This is known as a "dilutional hyponatraemia" which disappears with the diuresis that occurs about the 4th–6th day after operation. It should not be regarded as evidence of sodium loss.

Clinical Sodium Syndromes (Table 6)

Alterations in the normal homeostatic mechanism for sodium produce two types of changes—sodium depletion and sodium excess. These are roughly analogous to syndromes producing hyponatraemia and hypernatraemia respectively except that the plasma sodium may reflect not only a change in sodium, but also a change in plasma water. Accepting this, we will consider the changes in sodium metabolism as they are reflected in the plasma sodium, rather than total body or

Table 6.
Clinical Sodium Syndromes

Hyponatraemia
        Primary (Actual)—Sodium deficit
        Secondary (Dilutional)—Excess of non electrolyte fluid

Hypernatraemia
        Primary (Actual)—Sodium excess
        Secondary (Dehydrational) —Water deficit

exchangeable sodium, as we are faced so often clinically, with the need to explain an abnormal sodium level in the plasma.

Hyponatraemic Syndromes (Table 7)

A low plasma sodium may be due to an actual loss of sodium from the body and a change in total body sodium is also present. This is usually spoken of as a sodium depletion state, but in terms of the plasma sodium, we might regard it as a primary hyponatraemia. The corollary—secondary hyponatraemia, would therefore be that condition in which the plasma sodium is low, due not to a loss of sodium, but to accumulation of water—the low sodium syndromes.

Table 7.
Causes of Hyponatraemia

	PRIMARY		SECONDARY
a)	*Alimentary* Low Intake	⎧ Malnutrition	Post-traumatic
		⎨ Post-operative	Water intoxication
		⎩ Vomiting	Inappropriate A.D.H. Secretion
	High Output	⎧ Suction	Low Na-pump activity
		⎨ Fistula	Plasma expansion
		⎪ Ileus	Renal Failure
		⎩ Diarrhoea	
b)	*Renal*	Post -obstructive Uropathy "Salt losing" Nephritis Drugs e.g. Spironolactone	
c)	Endocrinel	Addisons Disease	

Primary (Actual) Hyponatraemia (Sodium Depletion)

This refers to the condition of loss of body sodium. The various ways or conditions which can produce it are shown in Table 7. Lesions of the alimentary tract predominate. The reason for this is obvious when one considers that the intake and out put of sodium (the external balance) is of the order of 100–200 mEq/day, whereas the sodium flux across the bowel wall from alimentary secretions is 5 to 10 times that amount, i.e. nearly 1000 mEq/day.

Loss of sodium is accompanied by loss of water, which at first keeps the sodium concentration in the E.C.F. constant. Later, as sodium loss outpaces that of water, the plasma sodium falls and some water passes into the cells to maintain osmotic equilibrium. The E.C.F. space is reduced and the fall in plasma volume leads to hypotension and eventually circulatory failure.

The patient has a dry tongue, but is not excessively thirsty—because he is hypotonic. The skin and subcutaneous tissues are lax and wrinkled, with loss of tissue elasticity and turgor. Inspection of the back should reveal no sacral oedema: if such is present, then the case is not one of sodium despletion. Intra-ocular pressure is low. All this is the picture of dehydration. The difference between salt and pure water loss is that the plasma volume is more rapidly affected, so that a weak rapid pulse and low blood pressure are quickly evident. Circulatory failure with collapsed veins, cold limbs and poor circulation will develop. With severe sodium depletion nervous symptoms of confusion and coma occur.

The haematocrit blood urea and plasma proteins are raised. The measured plasma volume is low, as is the plasma sodium (< 130 mEq/L), and chloride. Potassium concentration is normal. The urinary output is normal early on but becomes less especially when hypotension is present. The urinary sodium and chloride concentrations are low. The blood urea is an important measurement. A low blood urea means that sodium depletion has not occurred.

Treatment

Intravenous normal saline is required at a speed and volume dependent on the severity of the clinical state and the response to infusion. This is marked by improvement in circulation, or a rise in blood pressure, improved mental state, increased hourly urine output, and correction of the plasma and blood indices. It is better to judge the amount by the clinical response and urine output than rely on formulae such as: Sodium Deficit = 140 (plasma Na) × 30% of body weight. The 30% of body weight used to represent the E.C.F. but it is now realised that this is an excessive figure, 23% of body weight in adults is more correct. However in clinical practice if the above formula is used and is governed by clinical response with repeated assessment of the patient, all should be well.

If acidosis is present, sodium bicarbonate should be given. Normally one expects a metabolic alkalosis.

In severe salt depletion 500 ml. of hypertonic (5%) saline may be given to effect rapid replacement of plasma volume. One hopes that hypertonic saline may have the added effect of reversing the previous shift of water into the cells, thereby restoring, in part at least, normal tonicity.

Secondary Dilutional Hyponatraemia (Low Sodium Syndromes)

As already indicated, these syndromes produce hyponatraemia without altering the total body sodium. They can only do this by a process of dilution usually by excess water, but, as regards plasma level, by any non-sodium containing fluid which will remain in the intravascular compartment.

There are 6 main causes of syndromes.

1. Post-traumatic response:— Dilutional hyponatraemia may occur after any major injury or operation. The plasma sodium level is reduced to about 130 mEq/L. No treatment is required as it corrects itself by diuresis on the 4th–5th day.

2. Water intoxication:— This has already been dealt with on p. 18. It is in important and all too common cause, which must be corrected before serious cerebral cellular overhydration occurs.

3. Inappropriate secretion of A.D.H.:— This syndrome was first described by Schwartz et al (1957, 1960) in a study of two patients with bronchial carcinoma. The essential findings were a low plasma sodium due to water retention, a paradoxically high urinary sodium concentration, and a urine osmolarity above that of plasma. The blood urea is low even when the sodium output was restricted by corticosteroids, the hyponatraemia remained and only disappeared with simple water restriction. This suggested that for some curious reason, A.D.H. was being liberated. The increased urinary sodium concentration was thought to be due mainly to an increased glomerular filtration rate (Williams, 1963) and possibly to inhibition of Aldosterone release from an expanded E.C.F. volume. It is possible that the A.D.H. activity comes from the neoplasm itself as material with vasopressor activity has been recovered from a bronchial neoplasm (Barraclough et al, 1966). It is probable that this condition is more common and may be associated with other malignant neoplasms.

4. Low energy syndrome:— The hyponatraemia in this syndrome is thought to be due to an internal shift of sodium, i.e. into the cells, as patients are not improved by saline infusions but do improve when energy metabolism is restored to normal by improved nourishment. A simple example of such a syndrome is starvation, but it may be seen in any debilitating illness. It should not be confused

with the low sodium raised potassium state which may precede death, and for which there is no remedy. It is also important to exclude the other causes of hyponatraemia before deciding on energy deficiency alone as the cause.

5. Plasma expansion syndrome:— Infusions of non-salt containing solutions which may remain in the plasma volume for some time may cause a fall in plasma sodium. Intravenous glucose, fat, protein hydrolysates, mannitol, salt-free albumin or dextrans may all have a temporary and relatively unimportant effect.

6. Disease states:— Low plasma sodium is also associated with disease which results in retention of water. The prime examples are chronic congestive cardiac failure and renal failure, especially when discovered late and in which intravenous dextrose solutions have been given.

Hypernatraemic Syndromes (Table 8)

These, like the hyponatraemic syndromes, can be classified as primary or secondary, depending on whether or not the total body sodium is raised.

Table 8.
Causes of Hypernatraemia

Primary	Secondary
I.V. saline	
High protein high salt diet	Dehydration
Aldosteronism	
Cushing's syndrome	

Primary (*Actual*) *Hypernatraemia* (Sodium Excess)

Retention of sodium may occur along with water, as in cardiac failure, producing not hypernatraemia, but peripheral oedema. As the total body sodium is raised this is a sodium excess syndrome. But as the plasma sodium is not raised it does not properly fall into the group of primary hypernatraemia.

Sodium retention in excess of water does occur, and is unfortunately not a rarity in surgical patients. It is recognised by an elevated plasma sodium in the absence of dehydration. The hyperosmolarity produced can severely affect the brain, especially in children.

Increased salt intake over that of water is iatrogenically produced and is seen most commonly in 3 groups of patients:— children; those with neurological disorders; and patients receiving isotonic and hypertonic saline intravenously.

Infants may be given more sodium containing solutions by mouth, nasogastric tube, or intravenously than the kidneys are able to deal with. Excessive intake is also sometimes seen in unconscious patients and is liable to produce hypernatraemia, especially if accompanied by a high protein diet.

Hypernatraemia is also seen in neurosurgical cases in whom it was termed cerebral salt retention. In some of these patients there may be failure of the thirst mechanism which should limit salt intake and encourage that of water. In most cases, however, dehydration is the most probable cause of the hypernatraemia in these patients. Hypernatraemia is also seen in patients on excessive doses of corticosteroids or with adrenal overactivity as in Cushing's syndrome.

The main symptoms are due to pulmonary oedema, i.e. breathlessness and a frothy sputum with progression to circulatory collapse. In the neurosurgical cases especially cerebral confusion, apathy, convulsions and coma may occur. A close correlation between convulsions and plasma sodium levels was found by Morris-Jones et al, 1967. The incidence of convulsions was 10% when the plasma sodium was 140–158 mEq/L, and when the levels rose above this, the incidence of convulsions rose to 70%.

The haemoglobin and haematocrit are usually normal unless dehydration is present. The levels of sodium and chloride in the plasma are raised, that of potassium is normal unless Aldosteronism is present. The urinary output is high with raised excretion of sodium and chloride.

Treatment

The cause must be eliminated or treated. Water by mouth or intravenous 5% glucose will dilute the plasma sodium. The Aldosterone blocking agent (Spironolactone) may be used in particular cases.

Secondary Hypernatraemia—Dehydration

This is given prominence because for long, the hypernatraemia seen in neurosurgical wards, was thought to be due to some curious form of salt retention associated with brain damage—cerebral salt retention. The commonest cause is now acknowledged to be dehydration. The diagnosis and treatment is as for dehydration.

Potassium

This is the major intracellular cation with a concentration about 30 times greater than that in the plasma. The differential is maintained by the activity of the cell membrane. If this activity weakens due to lack of energy, injury, or death of the cell, there is a shift of potassium out of the cell and sodium enters it.

This difference in potassium concentration in the I.C.F. and the E.C.F. is emphasised by a curious and important dissociation in its control. There is practically no relationship in the concentration of potassium plasma in the cell and in the plasma, so that a deficit of potassium may exist in one compartment with a normal concentration or even excess, in the other. For example, in renal failure, a high plasma potassium may exist with a low intracellular potassium. Plasma levels reflect the concentration in the plasma at that point of time, and nothing more. It is nevertheless important as a low plasma concentration may not support life, whereas a high level is very dangerous and may stop the heart.

Potassium is required for normal cellular activity, in particular, that of cell enzymes, especially those involved in the Kreb's cycle and in muscle contraction.

The basic relevant data on potassium is shown in Table 9.

Table 9.

Basic Data on Potassium

Composition—Body
Total body potassium	—	3700 mEq
Exchangeable potassium (Ke)	—	3400 mEq or 48 mEq/Kg
Intracellular (98%)	—	3340 mEq or 47 mEq/Kg
Extracellular (2%)	—	60 mEq or 1 mEq/Kg

Balance—Daily
Potassium intake	—	80 mEq/day
Potassium output	—	70 mEq/day—Urine
		10 mEq/day—Stool

Concentrations in:—
Body fluids	—	Plasma	— 3·8–5·0 mEq/L
		Cell	— 140 mEq/L
		C.S.F.	— 3 mEq/L

Intestinal Juices
Saliva	25 mEq/L
Gastric juice	10 mEq/L
Bile	5 mEq/L
Pancreatic juice	5 mEq/L
Small bowel	5 mEq/L

Control of Body Potassium

Control of body potassium differs from that of sodium in that intracellular metabolism is of first importance. The passage of potassium into the cell depends on the cell's requirement for potassium for normal metabolism, and the availability of energy derived from glucose.

As about 70% of body potassium is in the muscle cells, it is obvious that injury or destruction of muscle will liberate much potassium which must be dealt with by the kidney. Also, a large proportion of potassium is in organs with a large cell mass, notably the liver. The metabolism of the liver and the effect on it of various agencies may lead to electrolyte shifts. These have been quantitated and evaluated by Shoemaker (1968).

Renal Control of Potassium

The renal control of potassium is not nearly as precise as that for sodium. Indeed, the kidney's ability to conserve potassium is poor. Even in the presence of a potassium deficit it continues to excrete the ion.

Under normal conditions, the intake of potassium is about 60–120 mEq/day. Of this, about 60 mEq/day is excreted in the urine and about 10 mEq/day in the stools. If the intake rises, renal excretion will increase. If it falls, the output will diminish, but even in starvation, potassium output goes on, presumably because potassium is liberated by the internal catabolism of the body.

Most of the potassium in the urine is secreted by the distal tubules due either to the effect of adrenal cortical hormones or to the exchange of potassium and hydrogen for sodium. If hydrogen ions are few, as in metabolic alkalosis, potassium will form the major exchange ion for sodium with, therefore, risk of hypokalaemia.

Effect of Trauma

There may be an increase in plasma potassium for a few hours after major surgery or injury, and usually an increased urinary potassium excretion, as part of the normal metabolic response to surgery. The urinary potassium excretion is maximal in the first 24 hours and lasts for 2–3 days. As there is no intake in that period this reflects a negative potassium balance which is quickly corrected when normal dietary intake is resumed. Some of the excreted potassium must come from destroyed cells; the rest from the action of aldosterone on the distal renal tubules.

Clinical Potassium Syndromes

These, like the sodium ones, can be classified as primary or secondary according to whether or not there is a change in exchangeable potassium. Table 10.

Table 10.
Clinical Potassium Syndromes

Hypokalaemia		
Primary	—	Potassium deficit
Secondary	—	Shift into cells e.g. Alkalosis
Hyperkalaemia		
Primary	—	Potassium excess
Secondary	—	Shift out of cell e.g. Acidosis: shock

Hypokalaemia

This is, in effect, a condition of lowered plasma potassium concentration. The normal levels are between 3·9–5·0 mEq/L. Hypokalaemia exists when the value is less than 3·5 mEq/L. As already mentioned, the plasma concentration is not related closely to the total exchangeable potassium. We prefer, therefore, to think of primary hypokalaemia in terms of a loss of potassium from the body—a potassium deficit, and secondary hypokalaemia as a shift of potassium into the cells, thus lowering the plasma concentration without affecting the total exchangeable potassium (Ke).

Primary Actual Hypokalaemia Plasma Concentration ↓ Ke ↓

The causes of this are shown in Table 11. Simply stated, the 2 main causes are, low intake, or high output. A combination of these often exists, as for example, after operation when the intake is nil and the output is increased. Loss of potassium is by two routes:— gastro-intestinal (vomiting, intestinal suction, fistula, diarrhoea) and urinary (polyuria, e.g. diuretics).

Table 11.
Causes of Primary Actual Hypokalaemia

Low Intake	High Output
Poor diet: malnutrition	Vomiting or suction
Alcoholism	Intestinal fistula
	Paralytic ileus
Anorexia—any cause	Diarrhoea
After surgery or trauma	Ulcerative colitis
Low sodium diet	Diuretics
Potassium free infusions I.V.	Aldosterone: steroids
	Drugs e.g. carbenoxolone

The greatest danger of a low potassium state is its effect on the heart. This has been known since the early physiological experiments of Ringer (1883) who showed weakening and finally cessation of the frog's heart perfused with a solution very low in potassium.

In primary hypokalaemia the intracellular potassium will fall and when this affects the heart muscle irritability may develop with bradycardia and possibly a fall in blood pressure. The E.C.G. shows characteristic changes seen in Fig. 6. These include ST depression going on to T wave inversion; prolongation of the QT interval and a prominent U wave may develop. The E.C.G. changes are probably related more to intracellular potassium than the plasma concentration.

The change in muscle activity affects also skeletal muscles producing symptoms of weakness which may go on to paralysis. (A useful physical sign is the inability to rise from the squatting position without assistance.) Weakness of intestinal smooth muscle is thought to account for the paralytic ileus sometimes seen in patients with hypokalaemia.

Potassium deficiency may be accompanied by deficiency in calcium or magnesium. These may be detected at the same time or occasionally

ECG in POTASSIUM DISORDERS

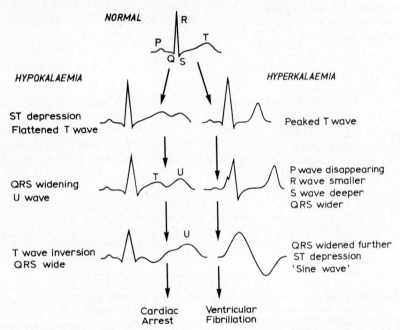

FIG. 6.   E.C.G. changes in potassium disorders.

become manifest when the potassium deficiency is treated, e.g. correction of hypokalaemia may be followed by hypocalcaemic tetany (Engel et al, 1949).

Secondary Hypokalaemia Plasma Concentration ↓ Ke—normal

In this, there is no real loss of potassium from the body but certainly there is a fall in plasma concentration. A shift has therefore occurred from the plasma to the cells. This is especially seen in alkalosis, in particular metabolic alkalosis. It must be emphasised, however, that not all patients with metabolic alkalosis have a normal Ke. In many, if not most, there is a loss of potassium in vomiting (10 mEq/L) and in the urine.

Diagnosis

By definition this is simply the finding of a low level of potassium in the plasma. This, however, gives no information of the volume of Ke or intracellular potassium. Indeed, Moore et al (1954), pointed out that not only could hyperkalaemia exist in the presence of a potassium deficit, but that it could be associated with toxic effects on the heart. The basic set-up is often the association of acidosis with potassium deficiency. For example, in diabetic acidosis, the plasma potassium may be normal or high even when the lean tissue mass is disappearing and a large amount of potassium is being lost in the urine. The "potential" hypokalaemic state is brought to light by the correction of the acidosis with sodium bicarbonate, glucose and insulin. Glucose moves into the cells taking potassium with it. Alkalosis will further aggravate the "potential" hypokalaemia as potassium moves into the cell, and increased potassium output may occur in the urine. Thus, in the correction of diabetic acidosis, potassium salts should be given even when the plasma potassium concentration is normal.

Apart from states of acidosis, it is rare to get a high plasma potassium concentration in the presence of a potassium deficit. The presence of a potassium deficit, i.e. low intracellular potassium, with a normal plasma potassium may be predicted as already stated by the E.C.G. concentration. Moderate potassium deficits may be present without changes in the E.C.G.

In summary, the diagnosis of potassium deficiency must be based on:—

1. History—Loss of energy—starvation

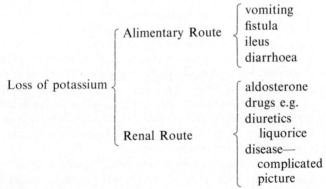

2. Investigation:

Plasma concentration
E.C.G.
Urinary potassium excretion—renal loss.
Isotope measurement—mainly research tool.
Tissue analysis—rarely used except in research.

3. In all consideration of potassium states, the Acid-Base state of the body must be considered.

Treatment of Potassium Deficiency

The treatment of potassium deficiency would appear to be simple and to consist of giving potassium chloride by the appropriate route—oral or intravenous. The problems lie in how much to give and how fast. The fact that the plasma concentration is related but little to the body potassium makes estimation of the deficit and multiplication of the deficit by a figure representing total body water an unreliable, even dangerous, exercise. The presence of other electrolyte abnormalities and changes in acid base state further serve to render the situation difficult.

As in all upsets in water and electrolyte metabolism, the speed of onset of the condition and its degree are all important in the speed and amount of replacement. In chronic potassium depletion, such as occurs in starvation, steatorrhoea, use of laxatives or diuretics, etc., potassium supplementation may be given by mouth as effervescent potassium tablets or even as Mist. Pot. Cit. (N.F.). If the degree of depletion is such as to cause cardiac embarassment, potassium chloride is necessary intravenously at a rate of 20 mEq/hour until the E.C.G. improves and the plasma concentration rises. Adequate renal functions is a safeguard against potassium intoxication.

When alkalosis is present, potassium chloride should be given in saline but in dehydration or when acidosis is present, the potassium is given in 5% Dextrose with insulin to assist in its transfer into the cells, or in an alkaline solution such as Darrow's. It is essential to proceed cautiously and not pass from hypokalaemia to hyperkalaemia just as one should not go from acidosis to alkalosis or vice versa.

In practice we find that in the severe mixed electrolyte upsets about 10–12 g (135–147 mEq) of potassium may be needed in the first 24 hours. Even this amount is only beginning to make up for the total deficit which in a moderate depletion state, may be up to 350 mEq in all, or 10% of total body potassium (Black, 1967) and in severe depletion, is correspondingly greater. These deficits should be replaced gradually to give equilibration in the body fluids time to take place and avoid sudden increases in plasma concentration.

Continuing losses of potassium should be calculated from the table data. Table 9. The main route of loss is renal and it is customary to give 40 mEq/day to cover this.

Hyperkalaemia Plasma Concentration ↑ Ke—normal

Whereas the previous discussion on hypokalaemia was complicated by the need to differentiate between the plasma concentration and total Ke. This is not such a problem in hyperkalaemia. The term signifies an increase in plasma concentration of potassium above the upper limit of normal (5 mEq/L). The total Ke is not affected as potassium in excess of that required, is eliminated by the kidney.

It is rare indeed to have a real increase in Ke and probably only in relation to infusion where too much potassium is given.

The various causes of hyperkalaemia are listed in Table 12. The most important and commonest cause is renal failure. Surgical Patients with: trauma and dissolution of body cells; infection, which increases metabolism and further tissue destruction; and renal failure, may show a very rapid rise in plasma potassium. This, the so-called hypercatabolic state, requires careful management.

Table 12.

Causes of Hyperkalaemia

Primary	Secondary	
Infusion stored blood	Renal failure	
Infusions of potassium	Diabetic	} Acidosis
Addisons disease	Shock	

There is really little clinical evidence of hyperkalaemia. It should be anticipated in the conditions stated and detected by measurement of the plasma electrolytes. The main effect of hyperkalaemia is on the heart. The E.C.G. (Fig. 6) shows enlarged pointed (tented) T waves which increases with the degree of hyperkalaemia until widening of the QRS complex appears and the rhythm becomes disturbed. The P–R interval is increased and the P waves disappear. Finally ventricular fibrillation may occur leading to death.

Treatment

This is basically the treatment of the underlying cause. Toxic levels of potassium, i.e. 7 mEq/L should be treated urgently and energetically to preserve cardiac function. The essential idea is to drive the potassium into the body cells until excretion can catch up with the raised plasma potassium level, or, until it can be removed by dialysis. Correction of the acidosis, if present, even to the extent of producing a mild metabolic alkalosis by infusion of sodium bicarbonate, will help greatly. This should be accompanied by infusion of 5% Dextrose and insulin. If renal failure is present with the need to limit fluid intake, hypertonic glucose may be used. But in these cases, haemodialysis would probably be best. Until this can be done, or in less urgent cases, potassium binding ion exchange resins such as Resonium-A (sodium polystyrene sulphonate) may be used in doses of 7·5 g four hourly by mouth or as an emulsion of 30 g as a daily retention enema.

Calcium

Most of the calcium in the body is present in the bone where there are two distinct fractions. A stable one which is intimately bound up in bone tissue, where movement of the ions in and out is slow. The other is labile and forms an exchangeable calcium pool of about 5 g in man. This is extremely small compared with the stable fraction which is 200 times greater (nearly 1000 g). Even so, being labile it is extremely important as a reserve to augment the plasma calcium. The calcium in the plasma is also divided into 2 fractions of approximately equal size. One is bound to protein with a small part complexed with citrate. The other is ionisable and diffusible for immediate use in the physiological activities of calcium. These comprise: bone formation, blood coagulation, and the function of muscle, nerve, and cell membrane. The relevant data for calcium is shown in Table 13.

Table 13.

Basic Data on Calcium

Composition—Body		
Total body calcium	1200–1500 g	
Exchangeable calcium	——	
Intracellular	1600 mg or 20 mg/Kg	
Extracellular	1500 mg or 20 mg/Kg	
Bone calcium	99% total calcium	
Balance Daily		
Calcium intake	0·8–1·0 g (approx. 10 mg/Kg)	
Calcium output	160 mg Urine (20%)	
	600 mg Faeces (75%)	
	40 mg Sweat (5%)	
Concentration in:—		
Body fluids—Plasma	9–11 mg/100 ml	4·5–5·5 mEq/L
Cell	80 mg/L or	4 mEq/L
C.S.F.	40 mg/L or	2 mEq/L
Intestinal Juices		
Saliva	0·5 mEq/L	
Gastric juice	4 mEq/L	
Bile	5 mEq/L	
Pancreatic juice	3 mEq/L	
Small bowel	4 mEq/L	

N.B.　1 mEq Ca = 20 mg Ca

To convert mg per cent to mEq/L divide by 2.

Control of Body Calcium

Calcium is present in the diet mainly in milk and milk products or as an additive to bread and other foodstuffs. Absorption is principally in the lower part of the small intestine with the help of Vitamin D. The presence of a large phosphate intake or steatorrhoea will render absorption defective. As calcium is present in the intestinal juices there is also an endogenous supply of calcium to the gut lumen for reabsorption.

Although the bulk of calcium is excreted in the faeces, the renal excretion of normally about 5–10 mEq/day is the main controlling mechanism for calcium homeostasis. Calcium is filtered through the glomerulus and is present in the tubular lumen in ionic form (90%), the rest is complexed with citrate. The amount filtered depends on the plasma calcium level. When this falls below 3·5 mEq/100 ml filtration stops; otherwise it continues uninfluenced by diet, in the beginning at least. After a month on a low calcium intake the output in the urine will fall. Reabsorption of calcium from the tubular lumen is dependent on factors still understood poorly. Certainly Vitamin D has an effect as a deficiency of this will reduce calcium excretion and excess of it will increase excretion. Parathormone has a like effect. Any factor which tends to raise the plasma calcium, such as osteolytic disorders, will increase the urinary calcium excretion.

Hormonal Control of Calcium

Two hormones have an effect on calcium metabolism:— *Parathormone*. This single chain polypeptide is produced by the parathyroids and has as its main action, the liberation of calcium from the bone. A secondary action is through its effect on phosphate excretion. Parathormone diminishes the reabsorption of phosphate which is excreted along with calcium. Finally, parathormone increases the intestinal absorption of calcium. The production of this hormone is controlled by a negative feed back mechanism based on the level of plasma ionisable calcium.

Calcitonin. This was isolated by Copp et al (1962) from the thyroid gland. Apart from the parafollicular or C cells of the thyroid it has also been found in the parathyroid and thymus in man (Galante et al, 1968). It has an opposite and more immediate effect than parathormone in that it prevents or slows down the liberation of calcium from the bone and so stabilises the level of calcium in the plasma.

Clinical Calcium Syndromes

As in the other electrolytes, these syndromes can be classified as PRIMARY or SECONDARY according to whether or not there is an actual deficit of calcium in the body or in the case of hypercalcaemia, an increase in total body calcium.

Hypocalcaemia

The causes of this are listed in Table 14. In primary hypocalcaemia there is a deficit of calcium in the body due to failure of absorption, as in rickets and steatorrhoea and an increased loss as in prolonged immobilisation, etc. In secondary hypocalcaemia, the total body calcium is normal but the plasma ionisable calcium is lowered due to a shift of calcium into the cells. This is classically seen in the alkalotic tetany, due to spontaneous hyperventilation.

Primary hypocalcaemia affects principally the bones producing rarefaction and possibly fractures. Secondary hypocalcaemia is usually more acute, and, as it affects ionisable calcium, the neuromuscular changes predominate. In these, there is an increased excitability of neuromuscular tissues with paraesthesia of fingers and toes and spasms of the muscles which may go on to tetany. The irritability can be demonstrated by tapping the branch of the facial nerve in front of the angle of the jaw (Chvostek's sign) or by producing clawing of the hand when a sphygomanometer cuff is blown up to the level of the systolic blood pressure for 3 minutes (Trousseau's sign). The diagnosis can be confirmed biochemically by measuring the plasma calcium level.

Table 14.

Causes of Hypocalcaemia

Primary	Secondary
Rickets	Respiratory alkalosis
Steatorrhoea	Pancreatitis
Hypoparathyroidism	Citrate toxicity
Malabsorption	Hyperphosphataemia

In primary hypocalcaemia, the total plasma calcium is low. In secondary hypocalcaemia it is the level of ionisable calcium (difficult to measure) that is important.

Treatment

As in all disturbances the cause must be elucidated and treated. In the situation of tetany, calcium gluconate or chloride can be given intramuscularly or intravenously. About 10–20 ml of a 10% solution of the calcium salt is given, and repeated if necessary. Alkalosis may be corrected by the simple expedient of rebreathing into a paper bag. Primary hypocalcaemia may require calcium tablets over a prolonged period. Vitamin D is also valuable in doses of 50,000–100,000 units daily. But prolonged administrations may cause Vitamin D intoxication with consequent renal damage. Table 15.

Table 15.

Causes of Hypercalcaemia

Primary	Secondary
Milk-alkali syndrome	Hyperparathyroidism
Vitamin D intoxication	Carcinomatosis
	Sarcoidosis
	Myelomatosis
	Hyperthyroidism

Hypercalcaemia Plasma Concentration ↑

Primary hypercalcaemia associated with a raised total body calcium, is very rare, as any increase in calcium by mouth is excreted in the stools, and parenteral calcium, in any amount, is seldom given. The most important and clinically most interesting cause of secondary hypercalcaemia, is hyperparathyroidism. Here, the plasma calcium is raised but as calcium is excreted in excess in the urine, the total body calcium falls. The clinical picture depends on a balance of intake of calcium, absorption, relative hyperactivity of the parathyroid, and excretion. Gross imbalance results in bone decalcification, patchy at first, but later more diffuse. Nephrocalcinosis, renal stones, and possibly even gallstones may develop. The abstraction of calcium from the bones results in a high level in the plasma. This is the lynch pin of diagnosis. Unfortunately, it is not always raised all the time. Indeed, there are occasions when only exploration of the neck will establish the presence of a tumour or hyperplasia of the parathyroids.

In the differential diagnosis of hypercalcaemic states, radiology and various laboratory techniques are used. The cortisone suppression test is sometimes helpful. Cortisone will usually depress the raised plasma calcium due to conditions other than hyperparathyroidism such as metastatic bone disease. Unfortunately, the test is not absolutely reliable as cortisone can affect about 20% of patients with parathyroid lesions.

Symptoms of mental depression, extreme lethargy, vomiting and coma dominate the clinical picture of acute hypercalcaemia. Rapid treatment is required to correct collapse, rehydrate patients who have been vomiting, and above all to lower the serum calcium.

Tachycardia, arrhythmias and persistent oliguria are danger signals.

Treatment

Haemodialysis and the intravenous injection of E.D.T.A. (ethylenediamine tetra-acetic acid) to chelate the calcium ions have been used but with limited success. Cortisone should not be relied upon for the therapeutic reduction of hypercalcaemia in disorders other than hyperparathyroidism as it acts too slowly.

Infusion of inorganic phosphates or sulphates have proved to be the most effective methods of lowering the serum calcium. Sodium sulphate acts by increasing the renal excretion of calcium and sodium phosphate by exceeding the solubility of calcium phosphate. Calcium deposition at the site of infusion may complicate phosphate infusions.

These methods of treatment have reduced the need for immediate neck exploration in acute hyperparathyroidism but exploration must be undertaken as soon as the hypercalcaemia is brought under some control as the results of prolonged conservative management are very poor. Utilization of the calcium lowering properties of Calcitonin may influence future treatment.

Magnesium

This is the second largest cation in the intracellular fluid and has an important role to play in enzyme activity. In this, it is involved in the functions of muscles and nerves as well as helping in the metabolism of carbohydrate and proteins. Recent interest has been focused on the deficiency syndrome, especially in intestinal malabsorption and on the importance of magnesium to the heart muscle. It is thought that magnesium ions are important for normal myocardial function and structure and when there is deficiency of them, oxidative phosphorylation suffers and structural damage to the myocardium ensues.

The basic data for magnesium is shown in Table 16.

Table 16.

Basic Data on Magnesium

Composition—Body

Total body magnesium	2500 mEq
Exchangeable magnesium	400 mEq or 6 mEq/Kg
Intracellular	360 mEq or 5 mEq/Kg
Extracellular	30 mEq
Bone (60% of total)	1500 mEq

Balance daily

Magnesium intake	25 mEq/day
Magnesium output	10 mEq/day Urine (40%)
	15 mEq/day Faeces (60%)

Concentration in:—

Body fluids —	Plasma	1·5–2·5 mEq/L
	Cell	30 mEq/L
	C.S.F.	3 mEq/L

Intestinal Juices

Saliva	8·2 mEq/L
Gastric juice	—
Bile	—
Pancreatic juice	trace
Small bowel	—

Control of Body Magnesium

This is still poorly understood. About one third of magnesium is bound to plasma proteins: the rest is freely diffusible. When taken in excess by mouth, magnesium is excreted by the kidney. In its absorption and excretion, it is governed by the same factors as govern calcium. Parathormone mobilises magnesium from the bone and increases urinary excretion. A curious feature in the distribution of magnesium is that while the concentration in the plasma is 1·5–2·5 mEq/L, that in cerebrospinal fluid is 2·5–3·0 mEq/L. The factors governing this differential concentration, not seen with any other cation in relation to C.S.F., are unknown.

Effect of Trauma

Following surgery, magnesium behaves in a way similar to nitrogen, in that there is increased excretion for 2–5 days (Walker et al, 1968). This, in the face of no intake, represents a negative magnesium balance.

Clinical Magnesium Syndromes

Hypomagnesaemia

This condition is rather uncommon, or at least, the diagnosis is seldom made. For years it has been a known complication of patients with advanced liver disease (especially in alcoholics) and in those on gastric suction and prolonged intravenous infusions (Flink, 1956). In the past decade or so, its occurrence with intestinal malabsorptive disorders and with intestinal surgery has been observed (Booth et al, 1963, Heaton et al, 1967). The underlying problem in this disorder, is that the clinical symptoms are rather vague so that its presence is unsuspected. Symptoms are, irregular muscle movements, twitchings, fasiculation, hyperirritability or convulsions, with or without psychiatric-type disturbances. When these occur in a patient with liver disease, alcoholism, intestinal disease or surgery, or one on intravenous infusions for a long time, then a serum magnesium should be done.

Treatment

Magnesium salts may be given by mouth or intramuscularly either as a test of cure or in the treatment of the diagnosed condition. Magnesium can be given intravenously in a dose of 1–2 g in 5% Dextrose. But, it is safer to use oral medication or intramuscular injection of 4 ml of 50% Magnesium sulphate. Unfortunately, the intramuscular route is rather painful.

Hypermagnesaemia

This is really very rare. The authors have never seen it although aware that it may occur when magnesium sulphate enemas are given to clear the bowel as in megacolon, toxaemias of pregnancy, and gastro-intestinal bleeding.

The symptoms are those of lethargy, muscle weakness, and C.N.S. depression.

Treatment

Calcium salts may be given intravenously to counteract the action of magnesium. In severe cases, dialysis should be considered.

Anions

Chloride

Chloride is the principle anion of the body, as sodium is the principal cation and with sodium, therefore, is largely responsible for the preservation of the osmotic pressure in the E.C.F. and water balance of the body. Losses of chloride from the body usually parallel those of sodium, but not proportionately, as bicarbonate can compensate for loss of chloride. This reciprocal arrangement is seen especially in upsets in acid base metabolism when a fall in chloride is reflected by a rise in bicarbonate and vice versa.

Chloride is involved in the exchange of oxygen and carbon dioxide in the red cells. In this, chloride passes into the plasma (chloride shift) and bicarbonate into the cells. This shift of chloride with oxygenation results in arterial plasma having a slightly higher concentration of chloride than venous. Chloride is also related to potassium in that a fall in plasma chloride is often associated with a fall in plasma potassium —hypochloraemic hypokalaemic alkalosis.

The relevant basic data for chloride is shown in Table 17.

Table 17.

Basic Data on Chloride

Composition—Body

Total body chloride	——	
Exchangeable chloride	2100 mEq/1	or 30 mEq/Kg
Intracellular	250 mEq/	or 3–4 mEq/Kg
Extracellular	1850 mEq	or 27 mEq/Kg

Balance—Daily

Chloride intake	100 mEq/day or 6·0 g Nacl
Chloride output	80 mEq/day—Urine
	10 mEq/day—Faeces
	10 mEq/day—Sweat

Concentration in:—

Body fluids —	Plasma	100–105 mEq/L
	Cell	8 mEq/L
	C.S.F.	120 mEq/L

Intestinal Juices

Saliva	10 mEq/L
Gastric juice	
Low Acid	60 mEq/L
High Acid	150 mEq/L
Bile	100 mEq/L
Pancreatic juice	100 mEq/L
Small Bowel	100 mEq/L

Control of Chloride Metabolism

This is similar to that of sodium in that the kidney is the main organ of control and chloride is reabsorbed with sodium in the proximal and distal tubules. Chloride may also be exchanged in the tubules for bicarbonate. A further source of chloride loss is in the sweat. This is normally very small, but at high temperatures, in the unacclimatised person, the loss may be considerable and occurs along with that of sodium. Tinkler (1966), found that the insensible water loss increased in patients having surgery in hot countries to over 2 litres and that in the unacclimatised, additional saline had to be given in amounts of 250 ml of saline per litre of infused fluid.

Hypochloraemia

This had been discussed also with hyponatraemia on P. 24 The disproportionate sodium to chloride loss is seen in pyloric stenosis when the concentration of chloride in gastric juice is so much higher than that of sodium, so that hypochloraemia and loss of hydrogen ions predominates with perhaps only a slight fall in sodium in the plasma. Hypokalaemia is often present in this condition and indeed, the mainstays of treatment are chloride, potassium and intravenous glucose to help combat intracellular potassium depletion.

Hyperchloraemia

This is much less common than hypochloraemia, occurring characteristically in uretero-colic anastomosis, in renal tubular acidosis, and rarely, as a result of excess administration of chloride. When chloride rises disproportionate to sodium, a state of acidosis is present. If the rise is proportionate, there is no appreciable change in pH. In uretero-colic anastomosis, the hyperchloraemia is due to an unfavourable ratio of chloride to sodium reabsorption from the urine held up in the bowel (Ferris and Odel, 1950).

Treatment of this condition requires the elimination of urinary stasis in the bowel, the administration of alkalinising salts and improvement of renal function by treatment of the renal infection (Lowe et al, 1959). Now that unreteroileal transplants are more common, the condition of hyperchloraemic acidosis is less common.

Bicarbonate

Although small in amount (24–28 mEq/L) bicarbonate ions are of immense importance in the body buffer system. Bicarbonate comes from 2 sources; ingested or infused along with sodium, or formed in the body by the hydration of carbon dioxide with carbonic anhydrase as the assisting elimination of carbon dioxide from the body and takes part in the renal tubular excretion of hydrogen ions.

The basic data is shown in Table 18.

Control of Bicarbonate Metabolism

Excess bicarbonate given intravenously is excreted by the lungs (70%) as carbon dioxide; the rest is buffered by the cells and excreted slowly

Table 18.

Basic Data on Bicarbonate

Composition—Body

Total body bicarbonate	——
Exchangeable bicarbonate	——
Intracellular	480 mEq or 7 mEq/Kg
Extracellular	360 mEq or 5 mEq/Kg

Balance—Daily

Bicarbonate intake	——	
Bicarbonate output	——	Urine
	10 mEq/L	Faeces

Concentration in

Body fluids	Plasma	24 mEq/L
	Cell	14 mEq/L
	C.S.F.	9·4 mEq/L

Intestinal Juices

Saliva	20 mEq/L
Gastric juice	——
Bile	35 mEq/L
Pancreatic juice	110 mEq/L
Small bowel	30 mEq/L

---

by the kidney. The level of bicarbonate ions in the plasma is maintained by the sodium/hydrogen exchange in the kidney. In this, sodium in the tubular lumen exchanges with hydrogen formed from the hydration of carbon dioxide. Both sodium and bicarbonate are then passed into the peri-tubular blood and E.C.F. If there is excess bicarbonate to hydrogen ions, bicarbonate is excreted in an alkaline urine.

Plasma bicarbonate is related intimately to the PCO_2: rising when it rises and vice versa.

Clinical Bicarbonate Syndromes

It is perhaps stretching semantics to classify the changes in plasma bicarbonate as syndromes, because they are really part of Acid Base metabolism.

Diminished Plasma Bicarbonate. A fall in plasma bicarbonate is seen in metabolic acidosis. In this, the change may be due to actual loss of bicarbonate as in diarrhoea or intestinal fistulae, or, more commonly, to the buffering of accumulated acids.

Increased Plasma Bicarbonate. This may be due to excess administration or to loss of acid as in hypochloraemic alkalosis. The metabolic alkalosis resulting has been discussed in the chapter on acid base metabolism.

Phosphate

This is the major anion of the intracellular fluid and forms an integral part of the protein structure of the body. Phosphates have many functions: they are linked to fat as lipophosphates and are active as enzymes, e.g. phosphatase; phosphate and calcium are related in their importance in the formation of the skeleton; they are important as cellular buffers and through the change of monohydrogen to dihydrogen phosphate, help to remove hydrogen ions from the body.

The basic data is shown in Table 19.

Table 19.

Basic Data on Phosphorus

Composition—Body

Total body phosphorus	—	600 g or approx 10 g/Kg
Exchangeable phosphorus	—	——
Intracellular		2000 mEq or 30 mEq/Kg
Extracellular		30 mEq

Balance—Daily

Phosphorus intake	1·2 g/day
Phosphorus output	Urine (60%) 0·7 g/day
	Faeces (40%) 0·5 g/day

Concentration in:—

Body fluids:	Plasma	1·5–2·3 mEq/L
	Cell	100 mEq/L
	C.S.F.	1·4–2·2 mg/100 ml

Intestinal Juices

Saliva	20 mg/100 ml
Gastric juice	——
Bile	15 mg/100 ml
Pancreatic juice	——
Small Bowel	6·8 mg/100 ml

Control of Phosphorus Metabolism

Phosphorus is plentiful in the diet being present in practically all foods and absorption from the gut is rarely defective. Phosphate is filtered by the glomeruli and about 90% is reabsorbed by the tubules. Vitamin D increases the rate of reabsorption; parathormone depresses it and increases the urinary phosphate and calcium excretion. The main factors affecting urinary phosphate output are: dietary intake (increased dietary phosphorus), increased output, acid-base regulation (acidosis increases phosphate excretion), and the endocrine system (parathormone and adrenal corticosteroids increase excretion).

Plasma Phosphate Concentration

Changes in plasma phosphate concentrations are not nearly as important as these in the aforementioned anions. A fall in plasma phosphorus is seen with renal tubular disease, hyperparathyroidism, and adrenal cortical activity.

A rise in plasma phosphorus is seen in renal failure and diminished parathyroid activity.

The Other Anions

These are proteins, organic acids and sulphates. The first two are important in body homeostasis, the last comes from the oxidation of the sulphur of proteins and while it rises in renal failure, is of little clinical importance.

Proteins

The plasma proteins are important as buffers and in controlling the passage of water from the interstitial space into the capillaries. Although the amount of plasma proteins in the plasma is large (about 7 g) this is only equivalent to 17 mEq/L, so the osmotic activity is small. However, due to their presence only in the intravascular compartment, this small osmotic activity has a definite importance.

Organic Acids

These are normally in small amount in the plasma and come from the metabolism of carbohydrates. Lactic acid is the predominant organic acid accounting for about 20% of the total. The others, pyruvic, citric, and acetoacetic acids are in very small amounts. In shock with low tissue blood flow and poor oxygenation of the tissues, these acids may accumulate to considerable amounts, particularly lactic and pyruvic.

REFERENCES

Water

Zimmermann, B. (1965). Pituitary and Adrenal Function in relation to Surgery. *S. Clin. N. Amer.* **45**, 299.

Wakin, K. G. (1967). Reassessment of the source, mode and locus of action of antidiuretic hormone. *Amer. Journal Med.* **42**, 394.

Sodium

Wardener, de H. E. Mills, I. L. H., Clapham, W. F. and Hayter, C. J. (1961). *Clinical Sciences* **21**, 249.

Wardener, de H. E. (1969). Control of Sodium Reabsorption. *Brit. Med. Journal* **3**, 676.

Walker, W. F. and Watt, A. (1967). The metabolic reponse to cardiac surgery. *Brit. Journal Surg.* **54**, 311.

Schwartz, W. B., Bennet, W., Curelop, S. and Bartter, F. C. (1957). Syndrome of renal sodium ion and hyponatraemia probably resulting from inappropriate secretion of antidiuretic hormone. *Amer. Journal Med.* **23**, 529.

Schwartz, W. B., Tassel, D. and Bartter, F. C. (1960). Further observations on hyponatraemia and renal sodiumion probably resulting from inappropriate secretion of antidiuretic hormone. *New Eng. Journal Med* **32**, 831.

Williams, R. T. (1963). Carcinoma of Bronchus with hyponatraemia and dermatomyositis. *Brit. Med. Journal* **1**, 233.

Barraclough, M. A., Jones, J. J. and Lee, J. (1966). Production of vasopressin by analyplastic oat-cell carcinoma of the bronchus. *Clin. Science* **31**, 135.

Morris-Jones, P. H., Houston, I. B. and Evans, R. C. (1967). Progress of the neurological complication of acute hypernataemia. *Lancet* **2**, 1385.

Potassium

Shoemaker, W. C. (1968). The action of epinephrine and other hormone associated with the stress response of potassium. *Rev. Surg.* **25**, 9.

Ringer, S. (1883). A further contribution regarding the influence of the different consitituents of the blood on the contraction of the heart. *Journal Physiology.* **4**, 29.

Engel, F. L., Martin, S. P. and Taylor, H. (1949). On relative of potassium to neurological manifestations of hypocalcaemic tetany. *Bull. J. Hopk. Hosp.* **84**, 285.

Moore, F. D., Edelman, I. S., Olney, J. M., James, A. H., Brooks, L. and Wilson, G. M. (1954). Body sodium and potassium III. International trends in alimentary renal, and Cardio-vascular disease: lack of c between body stores and plasma concentration. *Metabolisms* **4**, 334.

Black, D. A. K. (1967). Essentials of fluid balance. Blackwell Scientific Pub's. Oxford & Edinburgh.

Calcium

Copp, D. H., Cameron, E. C., Cheney, B. A., Davidson, A. G. F. and Henze, D. G. (1962). Evidence for calcitonin—A new hormone from the parathyroid that lowers calcium. *Endrocrinology* **70**, 638.

Galante, L., Gudmundsson, T. W., Mathews, E. W., TSE, A., Williams, E. D., Woodhouse, N. J. Y. and Macintyre, I. (1968). Thymic and parathyroid origin of calcitonin in man. *Lancet* **2**, 537.

Magnesium

Walker, W. F., Fleming, L., Sterart, W. K. (1968). Urinary magnesium excretion in surgical patients. *Brit. J. Surg.* **55**, 466.

Flink, E. B. (1956). Magnesium deficiency syndrome in man. *J. Amer. Med. Ass.* **160**, 1406.

Booth, C. C., Hanna, S., Barbouris, N. and MacIntyre, I. (1963). Incidence of hypomagnesaemia in intestinal malabsorption. *Brit. Med. J.* **2**, 141.

Heaton, F. W., Clark, C. G. and Goligher, J. C. (1967). Magnesium deficiency complicating intestinal surgery. *Brit. J. Surg.* **54**, 41.

Anions

Tinckler, L. F. (1966). Fluid and electrolyte observations in tropical surgical practice. *Brit. Med. J.* **1**, 1263.

Ferris, D. O. and Odel, H. M. (1950). Electrolyte patterns of the blood after bilateral uretero-sigmoidostomy. *J. Amer. Med. Ass.* **142**, 634.

Lowe, K. G., Stowers, J. M. and Walker, W. F. (1959). Electrolyte disturbances in patients with uretero-sigmoidoscopy. *Scot. Med. J.* **4**, 473.

3: Energy Metabolism and Nutrition

Energy

(i) Sources

The body is engaged continuously in the conversion of one kind of energy into another which is used by the cells to carry out osmotic, mechanical, electrical or synthetic work. The energy rich substances originating in the diet are glucose, fatty acids and amino acids which are partially broken down within the cell to form 2 carbon fragments (Fig. 7) which still contain most of the energy. These fragments are then joined to acetyl coenzyme A (Fig. 8) before any oxidation and further energy release can occur. Acetyl-coenzyme A is thus the final common pathway for the oxidation of carbons atoms from protein, fat and carbohydrate. Acetyl-coenzyme A combines with oxaloacetic acid to form tricarboxylic or citric acid and at the same time coenzyme A is set free. Citric acid is then converted back into oxaloacetic acid by a series of enzymatic processes and the chemical energy in the original 2 carbon fragment is released.

Energy is often required more rapidly than the tricarboxylic acid cycle can provide and the immediate demands are provided by energy rich phosphate esters present in the cells. Adenosine and creatine form esters with inorganic phosphoric acid. The most important of these substances is adenosine triphosphate (A.T.P.), which is present in all living cells. A phosphate radicle can be released from a molecule of A.T.P. very rapidly, liberating a large amount of energy and producing adenosine diphosphate. Some of the energy from the 2 carbon fragments which is being released slowly is used to reform A.T.P. by the addition of a phosphate radicle to adenosine diphosphate. Creatine phosphate also provides energy from its phosphate bonds for the recharging of A.T.P.

The high energy phosphate bonds provide a limited store of energy which is soon exhausted. If oxygen is lacking cells continue to function by anaerobic glycolysis in which lactic acid is produced providing enough energy to reconstitute A.T.P. When oxygen becomes available again the energy remaining in lactic acid is released by the further breakdown to pyruvic acid, CO_2 and water. The high energy phosphate cycle and the tricarboxylic acid cycle function simultaneously.

The body handles its energy requirements on a priority basis. The provision of two carbon fuel for the Krebs tricarboxylic acid cycle (Fig. 8) and usable energy has top priority. The supply of intermediate metabolites for the Krebs cycle and the maintenance of blood glucose comes second. The synthesis of body proteins while obligatory for ultimate survival has a lower priority. The storage of glycogen and fat take place only in the midst of a plentiful supply of energy sources.

SOME INTERMEDIARY METABOLIC PATHWAYS

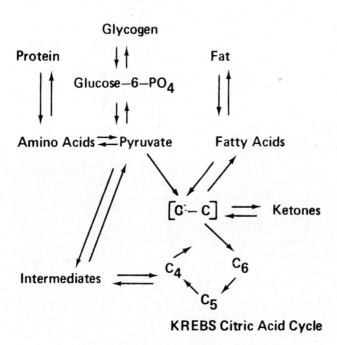

FIG. 7. Some intermediate metabolic pathways.

The organic and inorganic composition of the body is shown in Fig. 9. The body protein and fat stores comprise 40% of the body weight and the carbohydrate stores amount only to a few hundred grams which is present as glycogen in muscle and liver.

The actual needs of the body for nutrients are now known and many of the mechanisms by which food reaches the cells have been established. The ancient art of preparing and presenting food is now augmented by the precise and growing science of nutrition.

TRICARBOXYLIC ACID OR KREBS CYCLE (SCHEMATIC)

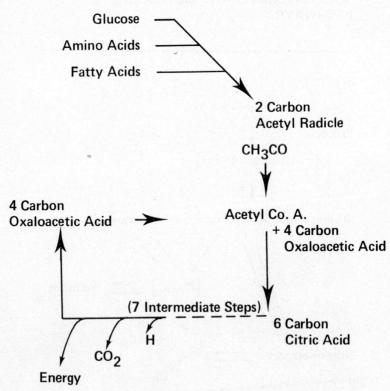

Fig. 8. Tricarboxylic acid or Krebs cycle.

The control of body weight in health is complex and involves a balance between the amount of food eaten and the energy requirements of the body. Body weight is maintained for long periods with daily fluctuations of less than $\pm 1\%$. The time scale for the regulation of the balance between energy intake and expenditure is periods of several days or even weeks as there is little direct relationship between the

food intake and energy expenditure on any day. The energy requirements are assessed poorly by means of the appetite and vary under
various circumstances. Activity, body weight, age, climate and pregnancy all influence the daily needs (Davidson and Passmore, 1969).

ORGANIC COMPOSITION OF MAN (70 KG)

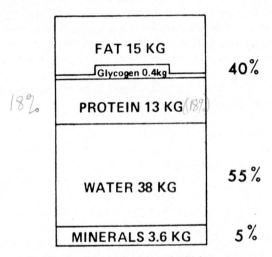

Fig. 9. Organic composition of a 70 kg man.

An estimate of daily requirements of calories and nutrients is shown in
Table 20 for resting and catabolic states.

Table 20.
Daily Requirement of Nutrients
per Kg. Body Weights

	Normal		Severe Catabolism	
Calories	40	(2800)	50	(3500)
Protein	1·0 g	(70 g)	2 g	(140 g)
Fat	1·8 g	(126 g)	2 g	(140 g)
Carbohydrate	5 g	(350 g)	6 g	(420)
Water	35 ml	(2450 ml)	40 ml	(2800)

Numbers in (   ) = Total for 70 Kg Man.

Surgical care frequently involves attention to nutritional needs. The
diseases for which surgery is required may produce nutritional problems

and chronic malnutrition will influence the response to treatment. Oral feeding is sometimes impossible for variable periods of time and artificial feeding is essential for survival under these conditions.

Requirements after Surgery

There is a prompt and significant reduction in body weight immediately after injury. The extent of the weight loss depends on the severity of the injury or operation and the presence of complications such as infection. As much as 10% of the body weight may be lost within 10 to 14 days of a major operation in a normally nourished patient.

The pioneer observations of Cuthbertson (1932) on post-traumatic nitrogen losses suggested that increases in energy demands and expenditure after injury or operation were responsible for some of this weight loss. It was postulated that tissue breakdown was necessary to provide energy for the greatly increased metabolic requirements of the body at this time.

Studies using direct calorimetry at the beginning of the century gave information about energy expenditure under varying conditions but the effects of trauma and surgery were not examined then. It was found that energy expenditure calculated by direct heat loss was in good agreement with expenditure calculated by indirect calorimetry using measurements of oxygen consumption, carbon dioxide production and nitrogen excretion (Atwater and Benedict, 1903). Kinney (1960) modified the method of indirect calorimetry to enable the resting metabolic expenditure of surgical patients to be measured easily. Samples of expired air are analysed at intervals and the gaseous composition determined. The excretion of nitrogen in the urine and faeces is also measured. These data and an accurate measurement of the intake of protein, fat and carbohydrate allow a daily calorie balance to be calculated and the metabolic expenditure estimated.

Using this method, Kinney (1967) has measured the changes in resting metabolic expenditure after various types of trauma and has found that elective uncomplicated surgical procedures are not associated with significant increases in resting expenditure. Multiple fractures are associated with increases of up to 25% and major complications, sepsis and severe burns may lead to increases of 40% in resting metabolic expenditure. All the measured increases in energy requirements after injury are smaller than might have been expected from the weight changes which occur. Fever often accompanies an increase in resting metabolism but Roe (1966) found no constant relationship between temperature and resting metabolism after injury.

Further consideration will be given to energy expenditure after injury when the metabolism of protein, fat and carbohydrate and the complete metabolic response to injury has been described.

Protein
Absorption and Utilisation

Protein is one of the major foodstuffs, essential for life. The contribution made by protein to the energy value of a normal western diet is around 15%. There is a constant demand for protein by the body due to continuous cell distintegration and renewal, particularly in the alimentary canal and bone marrow. This creates a demand which can be met from dietary sources only (Munro and Allison, 1964).

Proteins undergo hydrolysis by the proteolytic enzymes of the alimentary tract. Pepsin in the stomach is active around a pH of 1·2 and splits proteins into peptones and proteoses. The chief proteolytic enzyme of the pancreatic secretions is trypsin which is secreted in an inactive form and after activation acts best at a pH of around 8.

Digestion proceeds normally until amino acids are formed and almost all the ingested protein enters the body as amino acids. Proteins vary in their value as nutrients depending on their amino acid content. The function of amino acids is to maintain the structure of body cells and to provide raw materials for the manufacture of enzymes, body secretions, plasma proteins and haemoglobin. Amino acids pass from the intestine to the liver where the amino group (NH_2) is removed (Fig. 10) and goes to form urea. The remainder of the amino acid molecule is either converted into carbohydrate or fat or oxidised to CO_2 and water. Some amino acids cannot be synthesised by the body and have to be supplied in the diet (Table 21). Others, such as leucine,

Table 21.

Essential Amino Acids
and their Minimal Daily Requirements in Adults

Phenylalanine	1·1 G
Isoleucine	0·70 G
Leucine	1·10 G
Lysine	0·80 G
Methionine	1·10 G
Threonine	0·50 G
Tryptophane	0·25 G
Valine	0·80 G

lysine, methionine and tryptophan, cannot enter the carbohydrate pathways. Amino acids are the units from which proteins are formed and deoxyribonucleic acid (D.N.A.) and ribonucleic acids (R.N.A.) carry codes which arrange the amino acids within the cells in the correct sequence for the synthesis of different body proteins.

Nitrogen balance techniques are used to measure protein requirements and utilisation in man. Collections of urine and faeces have to be made over a number of days on a measured intake of protein. The use of food tables can give a reliable calculation of the nitrogen intake

(McCance and Widdowson, 1967). Most of the nitrogen is excreted in the urine and less than 10% of the dietary intake appears in the faeces under normal conditions. The amount lost in the sweat is variable and is normally about 0·5 g daily, most of which comes from desquamated cells of the skin.

PROTEIN METABOLISM

NORMAL

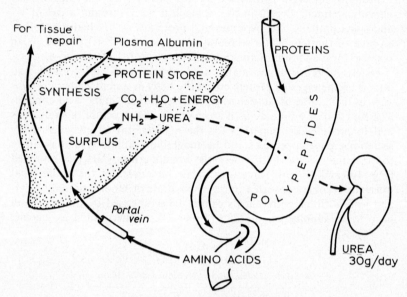

Fig. 10. Normal protein metabolism.

During growth a positive nitrogen balance is maintained which is controlled by growth hormone from the anterior pituitary. There is a sudden increase in protein accumulation at the time of puberty when the secretions of the gonads increase. Testosterone is a potent anabolic substance and its administration can produce retention of nitrogen. Non virilising analogues of Testosterone or anabolic steroids have been produced for clinical use. These substances will produce retention of nitrogen provided there is an adequate intake of protein but their application in surgical care is limited.

Dietary Requirements

The amount of protein required in the diet to maintain nitrogen equilibrium varies greatly. The nitrogen balance of a 70 kg man could be maintained by an intake of 45–50 g of good quality protein daily but 70–100 g is the amount usually consumed. It is recommended that adults should have at least 1 g of protein per kg body weight per day (Table 20). Very high protein diets can be maintained for long periods of time with no ill effects.

Proteins at one time were divided into two categories. Those of animal origin were called first class while those of vegetable origin were described as second class. This division is a little unfair as some vegetable proteins are but little inferior to animal proteins. Suitable mixtures of vegetable proteins can promote growth as effectively as milk proteins and merit the title first class. The nutritive value of protein depends upon the relation of the amino acids in its molecule to the amino acid pattern in body tissue. A deficiency of a single amino acid can render ineffective an adequate intake of an otherwise excellent protein. The amino acid composition of various foods consumed in this country have been calculated (McCance and Widdowson, 1967). Egg protein is very effectively utilised by man and supplementation of its amino acid content does not improve its biological value. Egg protein is now used frequently as a standard reference protein and rather than talk about first and second class protein it is preferable to classify protein by giving scores based on the ratio of the most poorly represented amino acid to the content of that amino acid in egg protein. The amino acid in any protein which is furthest below the corresponding amino acid in the standard is called the limiting amino acid. This is lysine in wheat and methionine in beef. The amount of any protein required to maintain nitrogen balance will thus depend on the amino acid composition.

The availability of individual amino acids has enabled studies to be carried out in man in which various amino acid mixtures were given and nitrogen equilibrium measured. Rose and Wixoin (1957), in a series of elegant studies have calculated the amino acid requirements of children, men and women (Table 21). Arginine and histidine are additional essential amino acids for growing children. These requirements are only applicable if adequate numbers of calories and non-essential amino acids are also included in the diet. The importance of calories in association with protein can be demonstrated by finding an increase in the urinary excretion of nitrogen when the calorie intake is reduced by 50% and the nitrogen intake unaltered. Each gram of nitrogen in the diet requires at least 200 calories for its most efficient utilisation by the body. This figure is only an approximation. The importance of maintaining this ratio is probably greatest when intravenous nutrients are being given.

The amount of protein in the body is variable and depends in part on the protein content of the diet. A sudden reduction from a high protein to a low protein diet is followed within a few days by a reduction in the amount of nitrogen excreted and equilibrium is again restored.

A return to a high protein diet is followed by a gradual increase in urinary nitrogen.

These changes in nitrogen excretion represent an amount of freely exchangeable or labile protein which the body possesses and this does not exceed 300–400 g. The body thus does not maintain large stores of protein above requirements. The reduction in the protein content of the body which follows severe injury is due to the destruction of cells and is not to be thought of as a reduction in body stores.

Protein Metabolism after Trauma (Fig. 11)

The importance of protein metabolism after surgical operation is recognised clinically and attention often paid to anaemia and hypoproteinaemia but the catabolism of lean tissue after trauma is difficult to appreciate and is frequently neglected. It is now almost 100 years since Bauer (1872) demonstrated that the concentration of nitrogen in

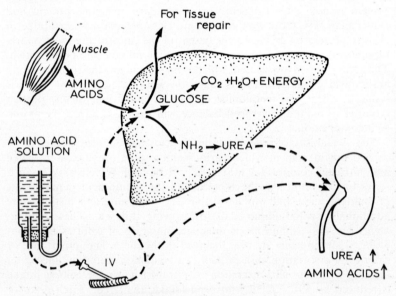

FIG. 11. Protein metabolism after trauma.

the urine was increased after a simple haemorrhage. Cuthbertson in a classic study (1932) observed that nitrogen appeared in excess in the urine and protein was broken down more rapidly than it is formed after fracture of a long bone.

The increased excretion of nitrogen in the urine after surgery is due mainly to urea, as much as 7% of the total body nitrogen may be lost after severe injury. The extent and duration of the losses depends upon the severity of the trauma (Moore, 1959). A man of average build may lose 400 g of wet lean tissue per day after a major operation. There is also an increased urinary output of all essential amino acids. Infused amino acids are utilised less effectively immediately after injury.

The rate of incorporation of amino acids into protein remains normal or is elevated after injury, suggesting that the rate of anabolism as well as that of catabolism is accelerated but catabolism predominates to account for the nett loss of nitrogen to the body (Levenson and Watkin, 1959). Blood urea also rises due to a combination of increased production and decreased excretion. Damaged tissue and disintegrating blood clot at the site of injury is responsible for some of the nitrogen produced.

There are two explanations for the breakdown of protein and mobilisation of amino acids after injury. Carbohydrate intermediates (Fumarate and Oxalate), are important for the tricarboxylic acid cycle and after injury their supply is threatened by an associated reduction in carbohydrate intake. Fatty acids although providing most of the energy output after injury cannot supply any carbohydrate intermediates. The infusion of fat emulsions after injury will supply carbohydrate intermediates and reduce nitrogen loss due to the presence of glycerol. It would appear then that the protein catabolism after surgery aims at providing carbohydrate intermediates at a time when exogenous carbohydrate sources are cut off.

There is some evidence also that after injury the liver is stimulated to synthesise more extracellular protein. This demand leads to the mobilisation of essential amino acids in muscle and other sites for transfer to the liver and the nitrogen in the urine may also reflect the deamination of amino acids carried to the liver in excess of the requirements.

The intake of food is restricted after severe injury or major surgery. The effect of the nutritional state and food intake before and after trauma on protein balance will be considered after a discussion of the effects of starvation alone.

Protein Anabolism after Trauma

The body restores the tissue it has lost quickly and an anabolic phase is reached about the fourth or fifth postoperative day when the balance of nitrogen becomes positive and as much as half the dietary intake will be retained and converted into muscle and lean tissue. The fat stores will be replenished during this time. The way in which this response associated with convalescence is controlled is not known. Insulin may play a part. Circulating amino acids are important and as these are liberated early in the response it seems that repair is initiated immediately after injury but only assumes a major role when the catabolic phase subsides. Growth hormone and thyroid hormone increase the rate of incorporation of amino acids into tissue but their role in the anabolic response to injury has yet to be defined. It may take two or three months for all the lean tissues lost in the response to a major injury to be restored completely and for full vigour to return (Cuthbertson and Tilstone, 1969).

The Serum Proteins

Separated plasma has a protein content of 7·3 g per 100 ml so that there will be about 230 g of intravascular protein in a blood volume of three litres, about twice this amount is probably present in the extravascular spaces.

Electrophoresis is the usual method of studying plasma proteins in health and disease. Proteins in solution have a negative charge and

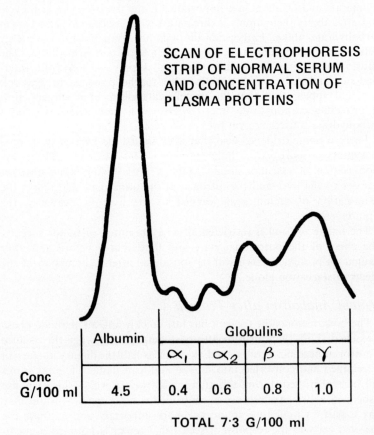

SCAN OF ELECTROPHORESIS
STRIP OF NORMAL SERUM
AND CONCENTRATION OF
PLASMA PROTEINS

	Albumin	Globulins			
		α_1	α_2	β	γ
Conc G/100 ml	4.5	0.4	0.6	0.8	1.0

TOTAL 7·3 G/100 ml

FIG. 12. Serum proteins.

move at varying speeds towards the anode. The composition of serum protein is shown in Fig. 12. The α, β, γ globulins are not separate substances but rather groups of molecules sharing similar ionic mobility.

Functions

The functions of the plasma proteins include the transportation of pigments, ions, hormones, and they are responsible for a small but important component of the osmotic pressure of serum. Albumin is three times as potent osmotically as globulin and a fall in the total plasma protein level to below 5·0 g per 100 ml may lower the osmotic pressure significantly enough for oedema to develop.

The plasma proteins provide a reserve of anions capable of taking up a sudden increase in hydrogen ions. This buffering capacity is less than 10% of the total buffering capacity of blood. Changes in plasma protein concentrations can alter the viscosity of blood.

Changes in Disease

Albumin is a single substance with a molecular weight of 80,000. Many diseases cause a fall in the serum albumin with a rise in globulin. A low albumin level may be due to defective synthesis in starvation, increased catabolism as after injury or abnormal losses of whole protein through the kidney or the gut or the skin after burns.

The α and β globulins include the glyco- and lipoproteins and the whole group is very heterogeneous with molecular weights of around 150,000. The α_2 globulins are synthesised in the reticuloendothelial systems and are increased after haemorrhage and trauma.

The glycoproteins are conjugated proteins containing carbohydrate. These substances are liberated by disintegrating cells and are therefore increased in the plasma after acute inflammation and tissue damage.

The lipoproteins are compounds of lipids and globulins which are firmly bound together and account for 75% of the fat in the plasma and contain neutral fat, fatty acids, phosphatides and cholesterol. The gamma globulins are a large group which can be divided into three sections, i.e., 1gG, 1gA and 1gM, and nearly all the immunoglobulins are found in these groups. Increased amounts are present in malignant disease, chronic infections and collagen diseases. The gamma globulins are a measure of host response to foreign substances.

The serum albumin, fibrinogen and many of the α and β globulins are synthesised in liver cells. The γ globulins are produced in the reticuloendothelial cells in extra-hepatic sites. Plasma proteins are synthesised from essential amino acids in the diet and different dietary proteins produce varying amounts of plasma protein. When protein is infused intravenously it enters the body cells directly. The ratio of turnover of plasma proteins has been measured and it was found that they can be replaced quickly in health. Half the amount lost in a moderate haemorrhage is replaced within 24 hours. The body contains about 500 g of albumin, the half life is 26 days and 12 g are normally resynthesised daily. A complete stop in the production of serum albumin would only produce serious clinical problems after 8–10 days. α and β globulins are turned over at twice the speed of albumin.

Changes after Trauma

Constant changes in individual plasma proteins occur after trauma. The level of the serum albumin falls slowly and there is an increase in α globulins. The fall in albumin is around 0·8 g/100 ml or 20% of the normal level and the lowest values are recorded between 4 and 8 days after injury. It takes about 14 days for normal values to be restored. The fall is related to the severity of injury and is maximal after major burns. The rate of turnover of albumin in injured patients is increased (Davies et al, 1969). The changes in plasma albumin are obligatory and are uninfluenced by nutritional supplies after injury.

The plasma α_1 globulin content is raised after surgery. The slow moving α_2 globulin which is not normally found in human plasma appears within 24 hours of injury and can be detected for about 10 days. The raised α_2 globulin in plasma 2 to 3 weeks after severe burns is reduced following exposure to warm dry air during the acute period.

The β globulins and plasma transferrin which constitute about 30% of the β globulin fraction may be increased significantly 10 or more days after a severe haemorrhage.

Plasma fibrinogen levels may double after injury, but patients with liver damage do not exhibit an increase. Serum mucoproteins and hexosamines are likewise increased. The individual proteins which are increased after injury, such as fibrinogen and α_2 globulin, have been termed acute phase reactants. The increase is related to the severity of the injury and both the synthesis and turnover in the liver are raised with synthesis in excess of breakdown (Owen, 1967).

It would thus appear that injury causes an increased anabolism or synthesis of some proteins with the appearance of an abnormal α_2 globulin and an increased catabolism of others. Much has yet to be learnt about the acute phase proteins.

The increased production of proteins by the liver after injury may be part of a feedback defence mechanism whereby the destructive lysosomal enzymes liberated within the cell by the stimuli associated with injury are inhibited and intracellular homeostasis is restored.

Fat

Sources

Fat is a most useful concentrated source of energy. It is present both in foodstuffs and in the fat depots of the body in the form of triglyce rides which are esters of glycerol and fatty acids, e.g.,

$$C\ H_2OCOR_1$$
$$|$$
$$C\ H\ OCOR_2$$
$$|$$
$$C\ H_2OCOR_3$$

where R_1, R_2 and R_3 are fatty acids.

There are a large number of different fatty acids available for triglyceride formation and fats are mixtures of different triglycerides. Animal fat contains large amounts of saturated fatty acids such as stearic, palmitic and oleic and small quantities of unsaturated fatty acids. Three of the unsaturated fatty acids, linoleic, linolenic and arachnidonic, are referred to as essential fatty acids, following work by Burr and Burr (1929) who demonstrated that these substances were necessary for the normal growth of rodents but their exact role in human physiology has yet to be established. The essential fatty acids are present in many vegetable oils.

The phospholipids are the next most important lipid component of the body fat after the triglycerides. They are present in the depot fat, the tissues of the body, the blood and form part of the cell membrane and are an important transport system in the body. Choline, ethano-lamine and serine are important phospholipids in human metabolism.

The sterols are another important group of biological substances all of which have a similar basic ring structure. Cholesterol is the principal sterol in the higher mammals and has an important role to play in the transport of fatty acids. Cholesterol is present in all food of animal origin, particularly eggs and animal fats. It is not an essential nutrient, however, as the liver is capable of synthesising it. Ergosterol is another important sterol present in many yeasts and fungi which is converted by ultraviolet light to Vitamin D. The precursor of Vitamin D in animal tissue is 7 dehydrotachysterol.

The average daily fat intake is around 100 g, 95% of which is absorbed even when daily loads of 150 or 175 g are given. (Frazer 1956.)

Digestion and Absorption (Fig. 13)

Most of the triglycerides in the diet are hydrolysed in the presence of bile by pancreatic and intestinal lipases either completely to fatty acids or partially to monoglycerides. Glycerol and the short chain fatty acids are water soluble and are absorbed by active transport. Fatty acids and glycerol are reconstituted within the intestinal cell to form triglycerides which aggregate in the lacteals of the small intestine to form chylomicrons most of which pass directly into the circulation by the thoracic duct. About 20 % of absorbed fat, particularly the short chain triglycerides, enters the portal circulation and liver. Some triglycerides are not hydrolysed and enter the body by being engulfed by the intestinal cell membrane by the mechanism of pinocytosis.

FAT METABOLISM

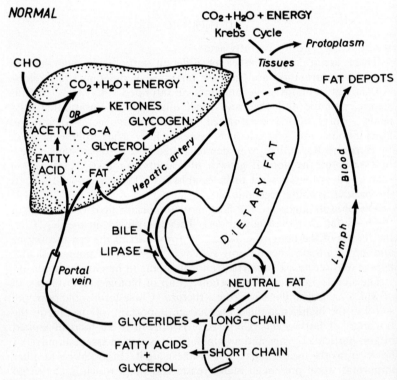

FIG. 13. Fat absorption.

Fat is carried in the blood as chylomicrons, low and high density lipoproteins and as free fatty acids. Fat in all these forms in the blood is always attached to protein. Apart from triglycerides, chylomicrons contain phospholipids, cholesterol and a small amount of protein. Chylomicrons are cleared quickly from the plasma by the action of tissue lipases. After a meal at which large amounts of fat are eaten the clearance rate of chylomicrons can be measured by estimating changes in the total serum lipids or triglycerides. The increase in serum lipids is maximal within 2 hours and normal levels are restored within

6 hours of the meal.   Infusions of intravenous fat emulsions are cleared from the plasma in a similar fashion and at the same rate as dietary fat (Carlson, 1962). The triglycerides which reach the liver are broken down and converted into fat specific to the species. The triglycerides formed in the liver are made up of fatty acids brought in the blood from the subject's own adipose tissue. Fat leaves the liver as fine particles similar to chylomicrons but very much smaller and also as low density lipoproteins which are complex collections of molecules (Fig. 10).

The lipoproteins in plasma remain as a metabolic mystery as they are altered but little by diet, exercise or injury. Most of the cholesterol in the plasma is in the B lipoprotein fraction and all the lipoproteins are concerned mainly with the transport of fat in various forms.

Utilisation

Adipose tissue receives fat direct from the intestine as chylomicrons, from the liver as secondary particles similar to chylomicrons, and as lipoproteins. The importance of carbohydrate in the laying down of fat has been emphasised recently. Glucose will enter the fatty tissues from the intestine and be converted into triglycerides. Adipose tissue is thus an extremely active organ with a considerable turnover. It has an autonomic nerve supply with nerve endings closely associated with fat cells and blood vessels. Triglycerides are being constantly broken down into free fatty acids which enter the blood to supply the energy needs of most tissues. The rate of deposition and mobilisation of fat depends upon the immediate energy requirements and supply of energy from dietary sources (Fig. 13). These rates are controlled by hormones and the autonomic nervous system but little is known of this endocrine control of fat deposition and utilisation.

Synthesis

The size of the fat stores varies greatly from person to person and may be as much as 20 kg in the too well nourished and as little as 1 kg in emaciated subjects. The fat content of adipose tissue is 85%, the protein content 2% and water makes up about 12%.

Triglycerides reaching adipose tissue in the circulation are broken down by the lipases of the cell membranes and the resulting fatty acids enter the cells for resynthesis into triglycerides. Carbohydrate is required in this process to provide an additional supply of glycerol. Fat is also formed in adipose tissue directly from circulating glucose and insulin is involved in fat synthesis by the body as it increases the rate of uptake of glucose by fat cells. Fat formation is sometimes increased greatly under physiological conditions, i.e. during pregnancy the stores may increase by about 4 kg in order to cope with the increased demands of the foetus and lactation. More knowledge about the mechanisms of increased fat deposition for physiological needs might help to unravel the problem of obesity in man.

Energy Release

The level of circulating free fatty acids in the blood is an index of the process of fat mobilisation for energy purposes. One molecule of plasma albumin can carry up to six molecules of free fatty acids. The level of free fatty acids in the blood under fasting conditions is low and not more than 0·5 mmol/litre. The levels are increased during fasting and exercise. Adrenaline, noradrenaline and growth hormone are known to increase the level of free fatty acids in plasma when injected. The role of the autonomic nervous system in the mobilisation of fat is important as nicotinic acid in large amounts blocks both sympathetic nerve endings and the plasma free fatty acid response to exercise. Growth hormone mobilises free fatty acids relatively slowly and by making energy available probably assists the deposition of amino acids to form proteins. Growth hormone levels are increased in the blood after exercise and injury and this response may have a part to play in the provision of energy in the injury period.

The amount of fat in the diet can vary considerably but about 40–50 % of the body's energy requirements normally come from dietary fat and a high fat diet is required for subjects burning over 4000 cals. per day. The oxidation of each gram of fat yields 9 calories. A high fat diet is essential for heavy manual workers but the more sedentary could well benefit by reducing their fat intake to about 20–25 % of their total calorie intake.

Response to Injury (Fig. 14)

The energy requirements after serious injury are increased and are met with principally by the mobilisation of body fat. The concentration of free fatty acids in the blood is increased immediately after injury (Mays, 1970) and is proportional to the degree of trauma (Birke et al, 1965).

Naftalin (1900) measured the total ketone content of blood at intervals after surgical operations and found that peak levels occurred within 12 hours. Similar peaks were only recorded 24 hours after starvation alone. These observations indicate that intermediary fat metabolism is modified considerably by the stimulus of trauma and as the carbohydrate stores are depleted rapidly, ketones and non-esterified fatty acids begin to be used within 12 hours of surgery and contribute significantly to the energy requirements at this time.

The importance of calorie homeostasis on the mobilisation of free fatty acids after injury has been studied by Carlson (1970) who found that large calorie intakes immediately after trauma led to a significant reduction in the levels of the free fatty acids recorded in the plasma. A reduction in calorie production and energy demands by maintaining the patients in a high ambient temperature also led within 24 hours to a significant reduction in circulating free fatty acids.

High levels of circulating free fatty acids have been implicated in the aetiology of fat embolisation of the lung, post perfusion pulmonary failure after cardiac surgery and cardiac arrhythmias. These occasional harmful effects of high free fatty acid levels have prompted attempts to reduce them and the blocking agent guanethidine is one substance which has been used experimentally to inhibit the sympathetic release of fatty acids.

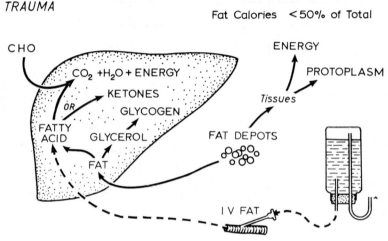

FIG. 14. Fat Metabolism after injury.

The lipoproteins in the plasma fall after trauma and low levels of cholesterol are observed within a week of severe injury. The rate of fall of lipoproteins follows a similar time sequence to changes in serum albumin concentration.

Plasma triglyceride levels do not alter significantly after injury but the rate of disappearance of chylomicrons originating either from the alimentary canal or from an infusion of fat emulsion is increased to keep pace with the increased demands for metabolic intermediates.

Carbohydrate

Digestion

Carbohydrate provides most of the energy in the average diet mainly in the form of starch and polysaccharides with small amounts of free sugars. The initial splitting of carbohydrates into disaccharides occurs in the upper part of the gastrointestinal tract. Salivary amylase hydrolyses more than half the ingested starch to maltose before it reaches the duodenum. Maltose, lactose and sucrose are the end products of carbohydrate digestion in the lumen of the intestine. Their further hydrolysis into monosaccharides (Table 22) is a function of the intestinal mucosa and takes place in the brush border of the columnar cells where the appropriate enzymes are situated.

Table 22.
Products of Carbohydrate Digestion

Polysaccharides	Disaccharides	Monosaccharides
	Maltose	Glucose + Glucose
Starch Glycogen	Lactose	Glucose + Galactose
	Sucrose	Glucose + Frucose

Monosaccharides

The monosaccharides are the simplest sugars. The principal hexoses, so named because they contain 6 carbon atoms, are glucose, fructose and galactose. Glucose as such is not present in many foodstuffs but it is the main constituent of starch. Fructose has the same formula as glucose but the structure is different and it rotates polarised light to the left and is therefore also called laevulose. Fructose is metabolised more rapidly in the body than glucose and insulin is not required for its utilisation. Galactose and glucose are the main components of milk sugar or lactose.

Sorbitol is a sugar alcohol (D Glucitol) produced by the hydrogenation of glucose and is present in small amounts in some berries. It is manufactured and used as sweetener in many foodstuffs and is prepared as a solution for intravenous feeding. Sorbitol is converted to glucose and fructose during absorption and metabolism. The pentoses or 5 carbon sugars are essential constituents of nucleic acids and their role as a source of energy remains uncertain. D ribose and Deoxyribose are widely distributed in cells and can be synthesised easily by the body. D-xylose is a pentose sugar found in food and is used as an index of intestinal absorption as it passes unchanged across the intestinal mucosa, is not metabolised, and is excreted unchanged in the urine.

Disaccharides

The disaccharides are the important dietary sugars (Table 22). Sucrose is split apart easily by hydrolysis during digestion to form glucose and fructose. Lactose, the main milk sugar, splits into glucose and galactose. Maltose after hydrolysis yields two molecules of glucose.

Polysaccharides

The polysaccharides which are of greatest importance in human nutrition are starch, glycogen and cellulose. Polysaccharides contain long chains of glucose molecules and are broken down during digestion to the disaccharide maltose and eventually glucose. Cellulose like starch is made up entirely of glucose but is insoluble and resistant to acid or enzymatic hydrolysis and has no nutritive value in man. Glycogen or animal starch is easily induced to liberate glucose. The liver contains over 100 g of glycogen which is used freely during starvation or after injury (Fig. 15). The other site for glycogen is muscle which contains over 200 g and this is a rapidly available source

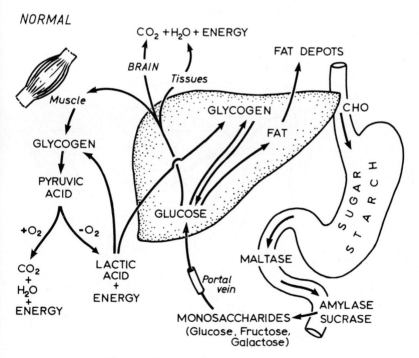

FIG. 15. Normal carbohydrate metabolism.

of energy. It can be used in a number of ways and may be broken down anaerobically when lactic acid is produced. When oxygen becomes available the lactate is oxidised to produce more energy. Some of the lactate from muscle work returns to the liver in the blood stream where it is resynthesised into glycogen (Fig. 15).

Utilisation

After digestion and absorption glucose may be utilised immediately, stored in the form of glycogen or enter the fat stores. Glucose can be used by all the tissues of the body and the central nervous system is dependent entirely on glucose for its metabolic needs. The demand is a continuous one as nervous tissue does not store carbohydrate and it is only under exceptional circumstances in starvation that any other energy source can be used by the brain.

The absorption of more glucose than the body can use or store as glycogen leads to the deposition of fat. However, there is evidence that even when the absorbed glucose is not in excess of immediate requirements a large proportion is converted into fat which is then utilised.

The level of glucose in the blood is controlled by a number of hormones. Insulin facilitates the passage of glucose out of the blood and into the cells of the body. Adrenaline releases glucose from the glycogen stores in the liver. Glucagon has a similar action and is

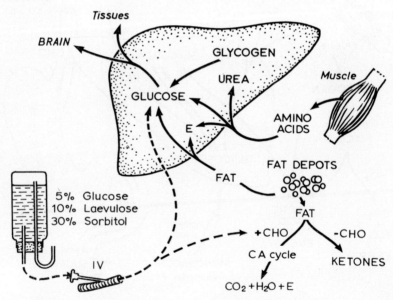

FIG. 16. Carbohydrate metabolism after trauma.

probably more effective. Glucagon assists the action of insulin by producing more glucose from the liver for transfer to the cells. The glucocorticoids increase the formation of liver glycogen and this in turn is broken down to produce excess glucose in the blood but this reaction is relatively slow.

When necessary the liver uses protein for conversion to glycogen and glucose, a process which uses considerable amounts of energy. It is thus essential that sufficient carbohydrates are provided in the diet to spare the use of body protein for gluconeogenesis.

Response to Injury (Fig. 16)

Following injury hyperglycaemia, glycosuria, a diabetic type of glucose tolerance curve develops as well as a resistance to insulin

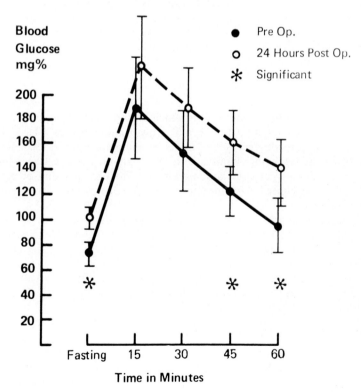

FIG. 17. Glucose tolerance before and after operation in six patients.

(Howard, 1955). The extent of these changes depends upon the severity of the injury and the term traumatic diabetes is sometimes used. The results of daily intravenous glucose tolerance tests after abdominal surgery indicate that the reduced tolerance to glucose lasts for about 3 days (Fig. 17). The rate of oxidation of glucose in tissues is reduced by 30% after injury due to inhibition of the reactions which allow pyruvate to be oxidised to CO_2 in the Krebs' cycle. Postoperative insulin levels in plasma are elevated both in the fasting state and at all times after the infusion of glucose (Ross et al, 1966). Reduced utilisation of glucose in the presence of an increased secretion of insulin indicates the activity of increased amounts of insulin antagonists like adrenaline and cortisol.

Adrenaline secretion after injury converts glycogen stores to glucose and provides an immediate and moderate extracellular carbohydrate reserve. Cortisol contributes to the hyperglycaemia by inducing gluconeogenesis in the liver where amino acids liberated in tissue breakdown are converted to glucose. Evidence for this effect comes from studies in adrenalectomised animals (Engel, 1955) and from battle casualties which showed a relationship between plasma amino acid levels and post-traumatic hyperglycaemia. Glucocorticoids in addition inhibit the peripheral utilisation of glucose and reduce the conversion of carbohydrate to fat. Local tissue hypoxia is probably another factor in maintaining hyperglycaemia.

Vitamins

Vitamins are organic substances which are necessary components of the diet and are required for normal growth and function. They are not used to provide energy but rather to maintain normal enzymatic activity. The intake of vitamins varies throughout the year, depending on the availability of fruit and vegetables. The ordinary diet of most people in the United Kingdom contains enough vitamins for normal requirements.

Clinical syndromes due to vitamin deficiency are never clear cut and are difficult to detect. The first evidence of a vitamin deficiency is biochemical and the tissue changes which are initially reversible occur later.

The sources and average daily requirements are listed in Table 23, and an important report on the subject has appeared recently (Department of Health, 1969).

Water Soluble Vitamins

Vitamin B Complex. This group includes thiamine, riboflavin, nicotinic acid as well as vitamin B_{12} and folic acid. Deficiency can occur from surgical causes as well as from a prolonged inadequate intake. Stagnation in the small intestine with bacterial proliferation produces

Table 23.

Vitamins	Sources	Average Daily Requirements
Water Soluble		
B$_1$ Thiamine	Yeast, wheat germ	1·5 mg
B$_2$ Riboflavin	Liver, milk, green vegetables	1·8 mg
Nicotinamide	Meat, vegetables	15 mg
B$_{12}$ Cyanocobalmin	Liver, fish, cheese	1 g
Folic Acid	Meat, vegetables	
C. Ascorbic Acid	Fruits, vegetables	75 mg
Fat Soluble		
A.	Eggs, milk	5, 000 I.U.
D.	Fish, milk, dairy products	
K.	Synthesis in gut	

a lack of B vitamins because the excessive bacteria consume the vitamins at the expense of the body. Subtotal and total gastrectomy may produce a vitamin B deficiency mainly due to a diminished intake.

Thiamine (B$_1$) is involved in the metabolism of glucose and formation of pyruvate. The interruption of this metabolic pathway will lead to cardiac and neurological abnormalities.

Riboflavin (B$_2$) is involved in hydrogen ion transport among nucleotides. When it is absent from the diet for long periods inflammation and desquamation of skin, particularly at the corners of the mouth, develop.

Nicotinamide is necessary for the action of several intercellular enzymes and when it is deficient scaling of the skin and pellagra occurs.

Vitamin B$_{12}$. The body stores of B$_{12}$ last for about 3 to 4 years. Patients who have had gastrectomy or resection of the ileum are liable to develop a deficiency.

Folic Acid. Folic acid is present in adequate amounts in the average diet and is contained in most green vegetables and animal tissues. Folic acid is also synthesised by small intestinal bacteria. Folic acid acts in conjunction with vitamin B$_{12}$ as coenzymes in the synthesis of nucleic acids in body cells. Absorption is defective in intestinal diseases associated with malabsorption and the demand is increased in the presence of chronic infections and malignant disease.

Vitamin C. Vitamin C or ascorbic acid takes part in tyrosine metabolism and in the conversion of folic acid to folinic acid. When it is absent collagen and osteoid formation is deficient. Haemorrhage occurs due to the lack of adhesion between the cells in the capillaries and the disintegration of fibrous tissue in the walls of small vessels. The most reliable indication of deficiency is the concentration of ascorbic acid in the buffy coat layer of centrifuged blood. Levels fall within 10 to 15 days after complete withdrawal from the diet but it takes several months for the ascorbic acid in cells to fall significantly and for clinical scurvy to develop. Patients with upper intestinal malignancy are often depleted of vitamin C before surgery. Vitamin C should be given in doses of 100 to 500 mg daily before and after operation until a normal diet has been resumed.

The demands for most vitamins rise after injury. The losses for example of Vitamin C in exudates may be considerable and large wounds and septic areas soak up Vitamin C rapidly. Lund (1941).

Treatment with Vitamins B and C in surgical patients has to be blind as there is no practical procedure for assessing the extent of any deficiency. Patients who are severely underweight at the time of surgery, patients with severe and prolonged sepsis, and those with severe granulomatous disease of the small bowel and colon should have parenteral administration of Vitamins B and C.

Water soluble vitamins are used liberally in surgical patients and little harm results from their overuse.

Fat Soluble Vitamins

Vitamin A is synthesised in the cells of the small intestine from carotene and is responsible for the health of epithelial cells. When it is absent, squamous metaplasia develops with blockage of sebaceous glands and follicular keratitis occurs. As Vitamin A is fat soluble lack of it will occur in patients with steatorrhoea. Disorders due to Vitamin A lack are rare in surgical patients.

Vitamin D facilitates the jejunal absorption of calcium from the diet and is necessary for the formation of normal bone. Vitamin D also facilitates the absorption of phosphate from the gut. Vitamin D deficiency is difficult to confirm clinically. The normal active adult does not need a dietary source of the vitamin and apart from the prevention of rickets in children Vitamin D is useful in the correction of low levels of serum calcium in patients with intestinal malabsorption or hypo-parathyroidism. Vitamin D in large and prolonged doses can be toxic and produce nausea, vomiting, polyuria and thirst. Irritability and depression soon follow. The level of serum calcium will be raised if overdosage with Vitamin D has occurred. A rise in serum phosphate after an intravenous injection of Vitamin D may be a useful test for deficiency of Vitamin D (Whittle et al, 1969).

Vitamin K is synthesised in the small intestine and it is doubtful if a dietary deficiency ever occurs. Malabsorption syndromes and obstructive jaundice lead rapidly to lack of the vitamin. Vitamin K is metabolised in the liver and is essential for the formation of clotting factors VII, IX, X and prothrombin. Synthetic Vitamin K (Menadione) is used for replacement therapy and daily injections of 5–15 mg will restore prothrombin activity within 2–3 days. It must be remembered that the intestinal antibiotics interfere with Vitamin K synthesis. Vitamin K is required therefore preoperatively in patients who have been starved as well as those with biliary obstruction and malabsorption.

Starvation

A reduction in the intake of food is usual after injury or surgical operation and is of little consequence for a few days as the body by its catabolism will supply energy but if prolonged then the sequelae of starvation develop. The response to starvation will be considered first in the absence of trauma.

Different organs in the body respond to starvation in different ways. The brain lives exclusively on glucose and requires about 130 g daily irrespective of the other needs of the body. The brain metabolises glucose completely to CO_2 and water, and a number of other organs rely heavily on glucose, for example, red blood cells, macrophages and fibroblasts demand about 30–40 g of glucose daily. These cells do not metabolise glucose completely and lactic acid remains. The lactic acid can be returned to the liver where it will be synthesised into glycogen by the Cori cycle (Fig. 10).

Fat is the main source of calories for many tissues during starvation, the energy being provided by free fatty acids or ketones from the partial oxidation of fat in the liver. The liver uses energy available from the conversion of fatty acids into ketone bodies (acetoacetic and B hydroxybutyric acids) for the conversion of amino acids into glucose. Tissues like brain which normally uses only glucose may adapt during prolonged starvation and use ketones. This ability to reduce the demand for gluconeogenesis is a defence mechanism which ensures that protein catabolism necessary to produce carbohydrate intermediates is kept to a minimum.

The glycogen stores in liver and muscle are very limited and amount to little more than a 24 hour supply for nervous tissue alone. Glycogen stores are depleted rapidly in starvation but not exhausted so that some glycogen remains as a reserve for sudden metabolic demands. Glycogenesis commences very soon after an alimentary load of carbohydrate is absorbed and metabolised. Continuing starvation stimulates the release of a regular supply of amino acids which are converted in the liver into glucose. This mechanism provides for the continuing demands for glucose.

As starvation persists and the supply of calories and amino acids runs out individual cells lose their functions and organs with a rapid turnover of cells are the first to suffer. Liver cells fail to utilise fat and fatty infiltration within the liver cells results. The synthesis of albumin is reduced while the level of globulin is maintained. A plasma albumin level below 3·5 g/100 ml is strong evidence of a severe nutritional deficiency or liver disease. Intestinal cells suffer early in starvation and the absorptive capacity is diminished so that the sudden introduction of large amounts of fluids and nutrients into the intestine after a period of starvation is to be avoided.

The provision of even small amounts of carbohydrate during starvation can have an important protein sparing action. The brain can utilise infused glucose directly and gluconeogensis from amino acids is reduced with sparing of protein. Even 400 calories from 2 litres of 5% glucose will prevent the catabolism of 60–70 g of protein daily.

Nutrition and the Metabolic Response to Injury
Intake

A number of factors have been shown to influence the extent and the duration of the metabolic response to injury or surgery.

Major abdominal operation in previously well nourished subjects is associated normally with a reduced intake of nutrients for 4 or 5 days at a time when the basal metabolic expenditure is increased slightly and the body is burning large amounts of endogenous fats and excreting excess amounts of nitrogen. There is no evidence that modest protein and calorie depletion at this time affects the rate of wound healing or the convalescence of the patient. There is also no evidence that the significant reduction in losses of nitrogen and body weight which can be produced by the intravenous infusion of calories and nitrogen is of any benefit clinically in the postoperative period in well nourished patients undergoing surgery of moderate severity (Abbott and Albertson, 1963; Johnston et al, 1966).

The contribution of starvation to postoperative negative nitrogen balance and the extent to which the nitrogen losses represent obligatory losses which cannot be altered significantly has been the subject of much debate. Almost all the negative nitrogen balance after trauma of moderate severity is due to a low calorie and protein intake and many workers have overcome the negative balance of nitrogen after surgery by infusing calories and amino acids. Wadstrom and Wiklund (1964) who were also able to reduce greatly the losses found that postoperative complications led to a further nitrogen deficit which they could not overcome. Johnston et al (1966) found that 47 calories per kg and 0·18 g nitrogen per kg almost completely prevented a negative nitrogen balance. These findings suggest that the catabolic reponse after moderate injury is small and is of the same order as the very modest increase in basal metabolic expenditure recorded at the same time. Spivey and Johnston (1969) in a study of the relationship between intake and balance in normally nourished men undergoing gastric surgery found that the catabolic response amounted to no more than 9 cals per kg body weight and 250 mg nitrogen per kg. The addition of these intakes to normal resting requirements in post-operative patients abolished the catabolic response completely.

It must be emphasised that in spite of significant reductions a pattern of rising urinary nitrogen excretion persists which is different from that seen in simple starvation. Maximal levels are recorded in the first day or two after starvation, whereas following injury peak excretion occurs on and after the third day.

Nutritional State

The initial nitrogen lost is mainly from labile body protein. The major loss comes from the metabolism of the lean tissue mass such as muscle. Labile body protein is a nutritionally dependent store so the nutritional intake before and immediately after injury will affect the nitrogen excretion. Patients who are underweight at the time of surgery exhibit a very minor response and such depleted patients can be kept in positive nitrogen balance by modest intakes (Fig. 18). The response

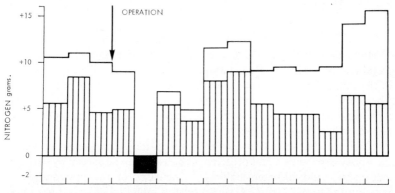

FIG. 18. Nitrogen balance after surgery in undernourished patient.

is less in women than men and the greatest responses occur in muscular youths. Attempts have been made to quantitate the changes in muscle mass after injury by isotope dilution techniques using creatinine but difficulty in achieving equilibration must keep this method in the experimental laboratory at the moment (Muldowney et al, 1957).

Severity of Injury

The severity of the injury is a major factor in determining the extent and duration of the response. Spivey and Johnston (1969) found that as the severity of the trauma increased, more and more protein was broken down and more and more calories and nitrogen were required to restore balance.

Soroff et al (1961) found that patients with severe burns required about four times their normal protein requirements to restore the negative nitrogen balance to normal with a very high calorie intake of around 90 per kg per day. These very high intakes are difficult to achieve even with the use of parenteral nutrients. Weight loss after major injury or surgery is thus inevitable because of the extent of the catabolic response and the difficulty of providing the large amounts required to restore balance. Postoperative complications, such as infection or venous thrombosis, will prolong the catabolic response.

Vascular Homeostasis

Rapid restoration of blood volume after injury is another way in which the catabolic response can be modified as hypovolaemia appears to be a potent stimulus for protein breakdown. Flear and Clarke (1963) showed that patients who were undertransfused at the time of surgery lost more nitrogen in the urine than those whose blood volume was maintained.

Environmental Factors

Major burns produce the greatest metabolic changes and increases in metabolic expenditure (Roe, 1966) due partly to the calories expended in the evaporation of water from the damaged skin (Barr et al, 1968). The evaporation of 1 gram of water requires 580 calories and the rate of evaporation depends on the temperature and humidity of the environment (Davies, 1970).

Careful studies have been carried out in patients after burns in which metabolic expenditure and protein catabolism were measured by indirect calorimetry and nitrogen balance. Increases in the environmental temperature from 22° to 32°C with a relative humidity of 20 % diminishes the excretion of nitrogen indicating that the reduction in calorie expenditure spared body protein principally (Davies et al, 1969). These changes may be due to a reduction in evaporative heat loss at high ambient temperatures.

Environmental control to diminish evaporative heat loss is now a most important aspect of the treatment of burns and its use in the management of other forms of trauma merits further investigation.

Cuthbertson and his colleagues (1968) have shown that protein catabolism following fracture of a long bone both in man and the rat can be reduced by a high environmental temperature. Evaporative heat loss is not an important factor in fracture patients so that environmental conditions must be modifying the response in some other way. The effects of temperature on the response to closed injuries is much less than after burns and no change could be detected during the first three days in patients having gastric surgery, nursed at 30°C and receiving varying calorie intakes (Spivey and Johnston, 1969). When compared with control patients nursed at 22–24°C.

Significance of the Metabolic Response

The modification of the response by increased intakes of nitrogen and calories by the control of the environment and by maintenance of blood volume challenges the concept of fixed obligatory changes following trauma which lead to inactive attitudes in monitoring and management of the injured.

Protein, fat and carbohydrate metabolism are all linked in a complicated manner both under normal conditions and after injury. The body needs glucose rapidly after injury at a time when normally none is available from the gut (Fig. 16). Protein catabolism is a rapid and efficient method of producing carbohydrate intermediates for use in the tricarboxylic acid cycle. Fatty acids are an inefficient supply of carbohydrate intermediates at any time and it is more appropriate that they should be metabolised completely to fill the energy gap left by the diminished intake and excessive demands.

The metabolic response once it has been evoked proceeds without significant or detectable control mechanisms and is therefore in a sense obligatory. However, it can be modified somewhat by the provision of nutrients and calories, maintenance of blood volume and control of the environment.

Ionic Aspects of the Response to Injury

It is not possible to consider the metabolic response without paying attention to the ionic fluxes which follow trauma and have been mentioned in Chapter II.

Potassium

The output of potassium in the urine is raised after injury and the peak excretion occurs within the first 24 hours when 70 to 90 mEq may be lost. The increased output lasts for two to three days and a positive potassium balance is restored several days before nitrogen balance returns to normal.

This disproportionate loss of potassium over nitrogen suggests a brisk exchange of cell base, the potassium being replaced by hydrogen or sodium after injury and being excreted with cell water. The plasma potassium level rises slightly after injury due to a shift across cell membranes. The tissue losing most potassium as well as nitogrogen after injury is skeletal muscle. After very severe injury the skeletal muscle may be depleted by as much as 30% as determined by a number of parameters including exchangeable potassium. Further sources of potassium are destroyed red cells and leakage from other damaged cells at the site of injury.

The control of this potassium loss is not usually a problem if oral feeding is resumed within a few days. However, if a normal intake is not restored and additional losses are present from the alimentary tract, then a significant deficit may develop quickly and may be of the order of 250–350 mEq of K^+. The infusion of 40 mEq daily from the third day after injury can soon restore balance provided renal function is adequate (Chapter II).

Sodium

The excretion of sodium is reduced after trauma and very low levels of less than 10 mEq per day may be lost. The rate of tubular reabsorption is increased. Postoperative sodium retention was reduced significantly when large quantities were given intravenously beforehand (Randall and Papper, 1958). This evidence suggested that postoperative changes were more likely to be controlled by a reduction in the functioning extracellular volume or by a reduced blood volume than by any changes in pituitary adrenal function.

It must not be forgotten that there is strong evidence that the normal ability of the kidney to handle sodium and water is reduced in the immediate post-injury period due to the powerful action of increased secretion of A.D.H. This led to the practice of giving small amounts of electrolytes and fluid soon after surgery and an intravenous intake of not more than 2·0 litres with not more than 80 mEq of sodium is usual in the first 24 hours. This established practice of respecting the postoperative antidiuretic drive was challenged by Shires and Jackson (1966) who produced evidence that the functional extracellular fluid volume shrank out of proportion to measured losses of plasma or blood volume after injury. These observations led to the widespread use of buffered sodium solutions during and after surgery for the purpose of expanding the E.C.F. spaces and abolishing the response to injury. This recommendation has been criticised recently because the premise on which it is based may be invalid due to inherent difficulties in the measurement of the extracellular volume in acutely ill patients. This expansion policy has led in a number of ill and elderly patients to serious over loading and the conservative view of the capacity of the body to handle fluid and electrolytes after injury must be maintained.

The changes in chloride excretion usually follow closely those of sodium except that sodium retention is greater than chloride. After 4 or 5 days a sodium diuresis occurs as an essential part of the response.

Other Ions

Walker et al (1964) have found a fall in the urinary excretion of calcium following injury and the calcium changes were similar to the sodium retention. Urinary magnesium on the other hand tended to rise during the 2nd to 5th postoperative days and was similar to the increased losses of potassium and nitrogen (Walker et al, 1968).

Trauma if severe may temporarily alter acid base balance by the increased production of acid metabolites in anoxic and damaged tissues and by a reduced renal and respiratory capacity to excrete these substances. Anaemia and hypoproteinaemia will at the same time reduce the buffering capacity of the blood. Massive transfusion of citrated blood will lead to an alkalotic state when the citrate is metabolised and the liberated sodium combines with body base (Litwin et al, 1959).

The serum iron level and iron binding capacity fall after injury, especially if blood has been lost, serum transferrin also falls. This is probably due to the diversion of iron for haemoglobin synthesis or the sequestration of iron in the reticuloendothelial system.

Water Production and Excretion After Injury

One of the factors which lower the serum sodium after injury is the hypotonicity due to the addition of sodium free water.

The breakdown of body cells and the oxidation of protein within these cells can liberate cellular water into the extracellular space. The catabolic response in a well nourished patient is such that the breakdown of 1000 g of muscle will lead to the excretion of 100 mEq of potassium and 730 ml of intracellular water. It is not uncommon for up to 75 mEq of potassium to be excreted daily after severe injury and allowances have to be made for the presence of about 500 ml of water daily from such intracellular sources.

Another source of water in the postoperative period leading to hypotonicity is the oxidation of fat. Each 100 grams of fat which is oxidised will produce 100 ml of water as well as 900 calories. This water is completely free of electrolytes. Water released by any of these sources enters the body water pool just as if it had been ingested or infused.

These sources of water from the lean tissue cells as well as from protein and fat oxidation have important teleological significance as they represent a protective mechanism against dehydration after injury in the animal kingdom at a time when access to water may be difficult or impossible.

The absorption of water from the intestine is reduced after injury, particularly if ileus is present. Water loss through the lungs and skin may be excessive if respiratory distress or pyrexia occurs.

Apart from these factors affecting water metabolism after injury, a strong antidiuretic activity is induced after trauma by a number of stimuli, hypovolaemia and fluid dislocation being mainly responsible (Chapter II). Urine production after surgery is reduced and between 500 and 900 ml per day only may be excreted and the osmolality is high. If water is infused after injury the rate of excretion is reduced significantly compared to resting conditions. The body weight will rise and plasma osmolality will fall sharply in the face of aggressive fluid infusions.

Enzymes

Changes in circulating and tissue enzymes is another aspect of the response to injury. After local injury intracellular enzymes appear in the blood draining the injured part. This is part of the local inflammatory response. The cytoplasmic enzymes, glutamic oxaloacetic transaminase (GOT) and lactic dehydrogenase (LDH), may come from destroyed cells or from neighbouring intact cells with altered membrane permeability. Wroblewski and la Due (1955) have suggested that many of the enzymes in the plasma after injury come not only from the injured part but from cells in other organs, and the response to injury is a function of cell metabolism and excretion at sites distant from the injured part. Recently Clarke (1970) has shown that the levels of the enzyme creatinine phosphokinase are raised three to five-fold in the first three days after gastric surgery. The increase in this enzyme is not related to muscle trauma and appears to be specific to the injury. SGOT and SGPT levels were unaltered in the same patients.

Lysosomes are small droplet-like bodies which are visible within cells and consist of packets of enzymes contained within a membrane. There is controversy over the role of the lysosome which contains enzymes such as acid phosphatase and B glucuronidase in the response to injury. It was thought initially that these lysosomal enzymes played little part in the cellular reaction to injury. However, the rupture of the lysosomal membrane may be the initiating factor in cellular injury as well as in the metabolic response to starvation. Lysosomal enzymes can break down protein, polysaccharides and phospholipids, of various tissues completely during starvation. It is not certain whether the lysosomal membrane ruptures as a specific response to injury irrespective of the nutritional state of the animal at the time of injury. Further studies of intracellular enzymes in blood and organs may help in the further understanding of the initiation of the metabolic response to trauma.

REFERENCES

Davidson, S. and Passmore, R. (1969). Human Nutrition and Dietetrics. Edinburgh: Livingstone.
Cutherbertson, D. P. (1932). Observations on disturbances of metabolism produced by injury to the limbs. *Quart. J. Med.* **25**, 233.

Atwater, W. O. and Benedict, F. G. (1903). Experiments on the metabolism of matter and energy in the human body. *Bulletin* **69,** p. 76. U.S. Department of Agriculture.

Kinney, J. M. (1960). A consideration of energy exchange in human trauma. *Bull. N.Y. Acad. Med.* **36,** 617.

Kinney, J. M. (1970). Amino acid and glucose metabolism in injury in man. Ciba Symposium on Energy Metabolism in Injury. London.

Roe, C. F. (1966). Fever and energy metabolism in surgical disease. *Monographs in Surgical Science* **3,** 85.

Munro, H. N. and Allison, J. B. (1964). Mammalian Protein Metabolism. New York Academic Press.

McCance, R. A. and Widdowson, E. M. (1967). *Spec. Rep. Ser. med. res. Coun.* (London) **80,** 297.

Rose, W. C. and Nixon, R. L. (1957). The amino acid requirements of a man. *J. biol. Chem.* **217,** 997.

Bauer, F. (1872). *Z. Biol.* **8,** 567.

Moore, F. D. (1959). Metabolic Care of the Surgical Patient. W. B. Saunders, Philadelphia & London.

Stevenson, S. M. and Watkin, D. M. (1959). Protein requirements in injury and certain acute and chronic diseases. *Fed. Proc.*, **18,** 1155.

Cuthbertson, D. P. and Tilstone, W. J. (1969). Metabolism during the post injury period. *Advanc. clin. Chem.* **12,** 1–55.

Davies, J. W. L., Ricketts, C. R. and Bull, J. P. (1963). Studies of plasma protein metabolism in burned and injured patients. *Clin. Sci.* **24,** 371.

Owen, J. A. (1967). Effect of injury on plasma proteins. *Advanc. clin. Chem.* **9,** 1–41.

Burr, G. O. and Burr, M. M. (1929). *J. biol. Chem.* **82,** 345.

Frazer A. C. (1956). Fat Metabolism. Scientific Basis of Medicine Annual Reviews. **4,** 311.

Carlson, L. A. (1962). Deposition, mobilisation and utilisation of fat. *Acta chir. scand., Suppl.* **325,** 5.

Mays, E. T. (1970). The effect of surgical stress on plasma free fatty acids. *J. Surg. Res.* **10,** 315.

Birke, G., Carlson, L. A. and Liljedahl, S. O. (1965). Lipid metabolism and trauma. *Acta med. scand.* **178,** 337.

Naftalin, L. (1962). Blood ketone and plasma N.E.F.A. levels in the immediate post-operative period. *Clin. Chim. Acta.* **7,** 614.

Carlson, L. A. (1970). Mobilisation and Utilisation of lipids after trauma in relation to caloric homeostasis. Ciba Symposium. Energy Metabolism and Nutrition.

Howard, J. M. (1955). Studies on the absorption and metabolism of glucose following injury. *Ann. Surg.* **141,** 321.

Ross, H., Johnston, I. D. A., Welborn, T and Wright, A. D. (1966). Effect of abdominal operation on glucose tolerance and serum levels of insulin growth hormone and hydrocortisone. *Lancet,* **ii,** 563.

Engel, F. L. (1955). The roles of the adrenal cortex and stress in the regulation of protein metabolism. Recent: *Progr. Hormone Res.* **6,** 277.

Lind, C. C. (1941). Ascorbic acid and human wound healing. *Ann. Surg.* **114,** 776.

Abbott, W. E. and Albertson, O. (1963). Intravenous protein alimentation. *Nutritio Dieta* **5,** 339.

Johnston, I. D. A., Marino, J. D. and Stevens, J. Z. (1966). The effect of intravenous feeding in the balance of nitrogen, sodium and potassium after operation. *Brit. J. Surg.* ~~54, 438~~. 53 *885*

Department of Health and Social Security 1969. Report on the panel of recommended allowances No. 120.

Wadstrom, L. B. and Wiklund, P. E. (1964). Effect of fat emulsions on nitrogen balance in the postoperative period. *Acta chir. scand., Suppl.* 325, 50.

Spivey, J. and Johnston, I. D. A. (1969). The effect of environmental temperature and calorie-nitrogen intake on nitrogen balance in the first eight days after abdominal operation. *Brit. J. Surg.* 56, 380.

Soroff, H. S., Pearson, E. and Artz, C. F. (1961). Nutritional requirements in burns. *Surg. gynec. Obstet.* 112, 159.

Muldowney, F. P., Crooks, J. and Bloom, M. M. (1957). The relationship of total exchangeable potassium and chloride to lean body mass and creatinous excretion in man.

Flear, C. T. G. and Clarke, R. (1955). The influence of blood loss and blood transfusion upon the changes in metabolism of water, electrolytes and nitrogen after trauma. *Clin. Sci.* 14, 575.

Barr, P. O., Birke, G., Liljedahl, S. O. and Plantin, L. O. (1968). Oxygen consumption and water loss during treatment of burns with warm dry air. *Lancet* i, 164.

Davies, J. W. L. (1970). Protein metabolism in burned patients treated at different environmental temperatures. Ciba Symposium on Energy Metabolism in Trauma. London.

Cuthbertson, D. P., Smith, C. M. and Tilstone, W. J. (1968). The effect of transfer to a warm environment (30°C) on the metabolic response to injury. *Brit. J. Surg.* 55, 513.

Randall, R. E. and Papper, S. (1958). Mechanism of postoperative limitation in sodium excretion: The role of extracellular fluid volume. *J. clin. Invest.* 37, 1628.

Shires, T. and Carrico, C. J. (1966). Current status of the shock problem. *Curr. Probl. Surgery.*

Shires, T. and Jackson, D. E. (1962). *Arch. Surg.* Chicago 84, 703.

Walker, W. F., Watt, A., Morgan, H. G. and McCowan, M. A. A. (1964). The effect of operations of varying severity upon calcium and phosphorus metabolism in the elderly. *Brit. J. Surg.* 51, 783.

Walker, W. F., Fleming, L. W. and Stewart, W. K. (1968). Urinary magnesium excretion in surgical patients. *Brit. J. Surg.* 55, 466.

Walker, W. F. (1967). Acid base balance. *Brit. J. Surg.* 54, 452.

Wroblewski, F. and La Due, J. S. (1955). Lactic dehydrogenase activity in blood. *Proc. Soc. Exptl. Biol. Med.* 90, 210.

Clark, R. G. (1971). The effect of surgery on the plasma level of creatinine phosphokinase. *Brit. J. Surg.* 58, 304.

Whittle, H., Blair, A., Neale, G., Thalassmor, N., McLaughlin, M., Marsh, M. N., Peter, T. J., Wedzicha, B. and Thompson, G. R. (1969). *Lancet* 247.

Litwin, M. S., Smith, L. L. and Moore, F. D. (1959). Metabolic Alkalosis following massive transfusion. *Surgery* 45, 805.

4: Endocrine Aspects of the Metabolic Response to Injury

The endocrine system responds to the stimulus of injury by an increased secretion of many hormones, the extent and duration of the response depends upon the severity of the injury and the presence of complications. Alteration in the rate of utilisation and excretion of hormones after injury affects the amounts which can be measured in blood and urine. The relationship between the metabolic and endocrine response is a complex one depending upon many factors whose effects have not been defined clearly. Despite this, there can be no doubt that the endocrine response is important for normal recovery and convalescence.

Pituitary

This gland, the controller of the endocrine system, increases its production of hormones from both portions of the gland after injury. The anterior pituitary liberates adrenocorticotrophic hormone (A.C.T.H.) and growth hormone and the posterior pituitary produces antidiuretic hormone (A.D.H.).

Anterior Pituitary

A.C.T.H. levels have been found to be elevated in the blood immediately before and after elective operations, but normal levels are restored within a few hours (Cooper and Nelson, 1962). The levels of A.C.T.H. in plasma after injury are greatly in excess of those required to produce a maximal adrenocortical response. The pituitary glands of patients dying after serious injury are depleted of basophil cells suggesting the complete exhaustion of A.C.T.H. stores in the response to major stress.

Most anterior pituitary hormones are secreted in response to a negative feed back mechanism whereby increases in the secretion of hormones by the target glands inhibit the further secretion of the appropriate trophic hormone by the anterior pituitary. The hypothalamus is an important station in this negative feed back chain as it synthesises link hormones which reach the pituitary by way of the hypothalamo-hypophyseal portal system and stimulate the release of pituitary hormones. Feed back receptors are present in other sites such as the mid brain structures.

The negative feed back mechanism for pituitary-adrenocortical secretion is altered during and after stress, when there are simultaneous increases in both ACTH and plasma cortisol levels. The administration of dexamethasone after operation to produce very high plasma corticosteroid concentrations fails to abolish the pituitary adrenal response to injury, suggesting that mechanisms other than negative feed back must be involved in A.C.T.H. release after trauma.

Growth hormone secretion can be stimulated by fear, insulin and pyrogens apart from the normal components of injury. Serum growth hormone levels measured by immunoassay methods are elevated for 1–2 days after surgery. Although patients who die within a few days of serious injury have very small amounts of growth hormone in their pituitary glands suggesting that massive secretion has occurred, there is little evidence that the growth hormone response is a function of the severity of the injury. Growth hormone is clearly not required for either the metabolic response to occur after trauma or for survival because the metabolic response to hypophysectomy or to operations in patients with no pituitary function follows a normal pattern.

Experiments in animals indicate that weight loss and growth retardation which follow injury in young animals can be overcome by the administration of growth hormone from the time of injury. However, in man there is no evidence that the anabolic action of growth hormone can be utilised to combat the protein catabolism associated with injury and daily injections of human growth hormone did not reduce the negative nitrogen balance in patients after surgical operation (Johnston and Hadden, 1963). Growth hormone may play some part in the later anabolic phase of convalescence. Increased levels have been found in the serum more than ten days after surgery and an anabolic and nitrogen retaining effect could be demonstrated at this time following the injection of human growth hormone (Gemzell, 1962). This suggests that the rate of anabolism in early convalescence can be increased.

Sexual function fades immediately after injury; men lose libido and women experience amenorrhoea until convalescence is well established. The urinary excretion of aetiocholanolone and androsterone (metabolite of adrenal androgens) are reduced for up to a week after injury and a significant fall in plasma testosterone levels have also been observed (Matsumoto et al, 1970). The secretion of pituitary gonadotrophin is reduced following injury (Charters et al, 1969), returning to normal during convalescence. The relationship between the return of gonadotrophic secretions, the anabolic activities of the male and female sex hormones and the protein anabolism of convalescence has yet to be established.

The synthesis and release of thyroid stimulating hormone is under the control of a thyrotrophin releasing factor (TRF) produced in the hypothalamus. Release of TRF is related to the concentration of free thyroid hormone in the plasma. Free thyroxine levels in plasma rise immediately after injury but no marked change occurs in plasma thyroid stimulating hormone (TSH) concentrations although a small fall has been reported on the first postoperative day (Charter et al, 1969). The effect of injury on TRF levels has not been determined.

Posterior Pituitary

The oliguria which persists for up to 48 hours after haemorrhage or injury was observed first by Claud Bernard in 1859. Jones and Eaton in 1933 described the problem of post-operative oedema which occurred when physiological saline solutions were used widely for the rehydration of surgical patients. Coller and others (1945) soon showed that the problem was due to an obligatory retention of sodium by the body after injury.

Infusion of glucose solutions alone after surgery caused a dilutional hyponatraemia with neurological changes. It was soon established that the rapid mobilisation of antidiuretic hormone explained the relative intolerance of postoperative patients to solute free solutions. Cline et al (1953) found high levels of posterior pituitary antidiuretic hormone in the urine after operation. These observations of the impaired handling of water and sodium after surgery led to the cautious use of intravenous fluids in the immediate postoperative period.

Sodium and water are handled differently by the kidney after operation. Water retention is more marked than sodium and patients with diabetes insipidus undergoing surgery have a normal retention of sodium but show no retention of water. Moran et al (1965) developed a bioassay technique for ADH and were able to measure frequent changes in ADH levels in plasma with considerable accuracy. ADH secretion is influenced by various components of surgical procedures (Fig. 3). The induction of anaesthesia is not a strong stimulus. ADH levels are often raised in pre-operative patients due to the stimulus of fluid deprivation. Intravenous fluids will cause a reduction in ADH levels in plasma. The incision of soft tissues produces some elevation and blood loss is a major stimulus as is traction on abdominal viscera.

Verney (1947) in elegant experiments showed that receptors in ramifications of the carotid circulation transmit stimuli to the hypothalamic neurohypophyseal system. Antidiuretic hormone release is inhibited when tonicity is low and secretion is increased as tonicity rises. After operation, however, when plasma is often hypotonic and the urine concentrated the promotion of antidiuresis is paradoxical and unrelated to normal mechanisms of osomolality control. It would appear that plasma volume changes and associated deprivation of intake take precedence over tonicity control immediately after surgery.

Henry et al (1956) localised the site of the volume receptors in the vascular tree. Baro receptors are present in the carotid sinus and aortic arch and stretch receptors in the left atrium. Distension of the left atrium in dogs causes a fall in blood ADH levels and a diuresis which is abolished by blocking the vagus. When a distended balloon in the atrium is deflated there is a brisk rise in the levels of ADH in plasma. These findings offer an explanation for the dilutional syndrome which may follow the surgical correction of a tight mitral stenosis in man. The importance of nervous afferent pathways in the control of ADH secretion is emphasised by the observation that the ADH secretion induced by trauma in the limb of an animal is abolished by peripheral nerve section. The response to visceral stimulation can be abolished by appropriate regional or spinal anaesthesia. The afferent limb of the ADH control system thus originates in a number of sensors.

An inverse relationship between solute clearance and ADH levels in plasma was found to exist, suggesting that ADH depresses the solute bound losses of urine by changing either the glomerular filtration rate or renal blood flow. If it is necessary to increase urine output after surgery a solute load is required to saturate the ADH mechanism. The administration of modest amounts of sodium (75 to 100 mEq) is the most effective method of producing a modest increase in urine production and is a more physiological approach than the use of mannitol or urea.

Adrenal

The effects of injury and operation on the adrenal have been studied extensively. The adrenal medulla was at first thought to be the more important with its protective role after injury (Cannon, 1929) but Selye (1946) emphasised the importance of the cortex and postulated that it initiated and controlled the total response to stress.

The hormones of the adrenal cortex are most important in the maintenance of blood volume, the retention of salt and water and are essential for normal recovery. The secretions of the medulla have a powerful vasopressor activity which accommodates the circulatory system to any reduction in blood volume which might occur during injury.

Adrenal Cortex

The adrenal cortex produces three groups of hormones. The gluco-corticoids of which cortisol is the principal hormone and the electro-corticoids of which aldosterone is the most important are involved in the metabolic response. The sex hormones of the adrenal cortex are unaffected by trauma.

(i) *Cortisol*

The factors influencing the secretion of cortisol are shown in Fig. 19. Cortisol is released in response to adrenocorticotrophic hormone, the secretion of which is under the control of a negative feed back mechanism. The plasma cortisol level exhibits a diurnal rhythm and normally ranges between 2 and 24 μg/100 ml.

ADRENAL STEROID RELEASE

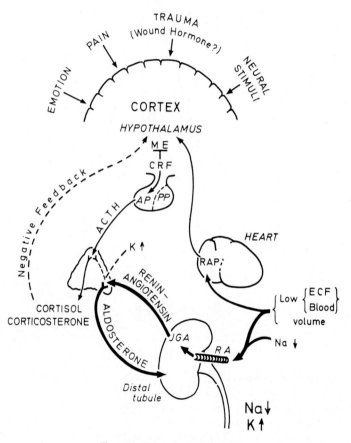

Fig. 19. Adrenal steroid release.

After injury there is a brisk rise in the plasma cortisol concentration which reaches a peak within 4 to 6 hours and returns to the resting level within 24 hours (Franksson and Gemzell, 1953 (Fig. 20). The level of plasma cortisol at any time after injury is related not only to increased secretion by the adrenal but also to diminished conjugation in the liver, many of whose functions are diminished after trauma.

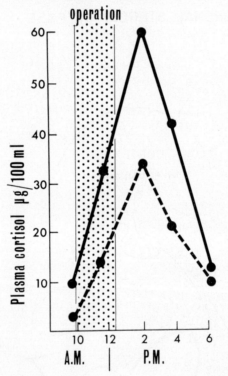

EFFECT OF MAJOR OPERATION ON LEVEL OF PLASMA CORTISOL (two patients)

FIG. 20. Plasma cortisol levels during surgery.

Reduced tissue utilisation and altered renal excretion are other factors which influence the plasma level. The finding of low levels in surgical patients is suggestive of adrenal insufficiency but isolated readings are of little value in view of the extent of normal diurnal variations and the many factors involved. Early increases in plasma cortisol levels after surgery have been found to parallel levels of plasma A.C.T.H. (Cooper and Nelson, 1962) so that the negative feed back mechanism must not be operating in the immediate post injury period.

Confirmation of increased rates of adrenocortical secretion after injury comes from the work of Hume et al (1962) who used an indwelling adrenal vein catheter to collect samples of blood during and after surgical operation in humans. They found that the secretion of cortisol was increased tenfold immediately after surgery (from 3·1 μg per minute to 30 μg per minute) with a fall to normal within 24 hours. The administration of A.C.T.H. during operation produced no further increase in plasma cortisol levels indicating a maximal response to the injury stimulus, but 24 hours later there was an immediate fresh response to a further A.C.T.H. infusion. The frequency with which the adrenal responds maximally to surgical stress depends on a number of factors and about 20% of patients undergoing operation of minor or moderate severity show no response. Hypotension is an effective stimulus for the secretion of cortisol and hypovolaemia stimulates secretion even in the absence of hypotension (Gann et al, 1965).

Cortisol is bound either to a plasma globulin fraction or is in a free form and normally only a small fraction of the total amount of circulating cortisol appears unchanged in the urine. With increased levels of plasma cortisol, the binding sites become saturated, and more free cortisol is excreted by the kidney. Measurement of the urinary free cortisol gives a more accurate picture of adrenocortical activity than any other method but the technique is difficult (Espiner, 1966).

The urinary excretion of cortisol metabolites usually measured as 17 oxogenic steroids is increased for 3 or 4 days after surgery, rising from 3 mg per day to 18 to 20 mg per day (Moore et al, 1955). Postoperative complications such as haemorrhage or infection prolongs and further augments the increased excretion of 17 oxogenic steroids. The output of urinary metabolites of adrenal androgens (17 oxosteroids) alters but little after surgical operation and may even fall (Tanaka et al, 1970).

Measurement of free cortisol in the urine in a group of patients about to undergo surgical operations showed levels comparable to those found in patients with florid Cushing's syndrome indicating the important role of fear and apprehension in controlling the activity of the adrenal cortex (Espiner, 1966). The range of response of urinary free cortisol to trauma varies widely and thirty to forty fold increases in the 24 hour urinary excretion were found after major operations like abdomino-perineal resection of the rectum (Fig. 21). Bilateral stripping of varicose veins produced similar results. Hernia repair and other minor procedures, however, produced no change, or only a small increase. These observations suggest that the extent of the adrenocortical response may be an index of the amount of tissue damage, haemorrhage or afferent nerve stimulation which has occurred during operation.

The actual cortisol secretion rate can be measured by the administration of C14 cortisol and collecting the urine for 24 hours. A specific metabolite of cortisol is then isolated from the urine, purified and the specific activity calculated.

The use of this technique confirms the extent of the response as measured by other means.

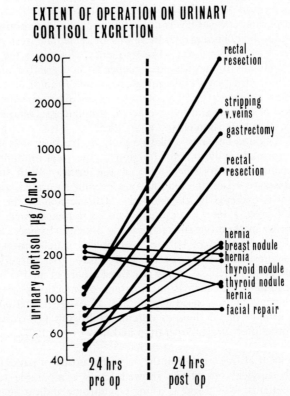

FIG. 21. Urinary corticol excretion after operation.

(ii) *Aldosterone*

The electrocorticoid aldosterone was isolated from the adrenal gland in 1952. The potent sodium retaining property of this hormone is certainly one explanation of the changes in sodium and potassium excretion following injury. Further evidence of aldosterone activity came from studies by Llaurado (1955) in which extracts of urine from injured subjects were assayed for aldosterone activity by injecting them into adrenalectomised rats and measuring the ratio of sodium to potassium measured in the rat urine. Increased amounts of an aldosterone-like substance were found in the urine of postoperative patients using these methods. Direct measurements have since confirmed that there is a brisk increase in the aldosterone secretion rate during major surgery (Hume et al, 1962) and urinary aldosterone levels remain elevated for a few days afterwards. Many factors control the secretion of aldosterone and after injury (Fig. 19) sodium depletion and hypovolaemia are probably the most important (Bartter, 1956).

Changes in aldosterone secretion are similar to those of cortisol and are related to the extent of the injury. Skillman et al (1967) used a double isotope dilutional technique demonstrating an increased aldosterone secretion rate following haemorrhage alone.

The importance of aldosterone in the postoperative retention of sodium has been demonstrated by giving an aldosterone antagonist (spironolactone) during and after surgery. Postoperative sodium retention can be reduced but not abolished by an aldosterone blocking substance, but the renal handling of potassium is unaffected. Kay (1968) confirmed that a blocking agent could not abolish completely normal sodium retention after trauma, so that aldosterone is not the only control of sodium excretion in postoperative patients, and cortisol may have its role to play in electrolyte balance after injury.

Peripheral plasma renin levels have been reported to be elevated during laparotomy (Blair-West et al, 1967) and the circulatory responses to trauma might well initiate the release of renin which in turn increases aldosterone secretion. Walker (1965) found that the careful monitoring of patients undergoing open heart surgery so that blood volume was never depleted led to a reduction in aldosterone secretion compared with operations where blood volume had not been maintained adequately. This study indicated the importance of volume receptors located in the right atrium and in the juxtaglomerular body in the kidney and re-emphasises the necessity for accurate maintenance of vascular homeostasis during and after surgery.

Although moderate increases in A.C.T.H. have little effect on aldosterone secretion, very high circulating levels augment aldosterone secretion and probably are important in the postoperative period. A raised concentration of potassium in blood can also release aldosterone. 5-hydroxytryptamine, which is released in injured tissues, has been shown to be able to stimulate aldosterone secretion.

Adrenal Medulla

Cannon (1929) suggested that the sympathetic nervous system and the adrenal medulla played an important role in the metabolic response to stress and the elevation of pulse rate and vasoconstriction associated with injury. A ten fold increase in catecholamine secretion follows major operations in man and an increased urinary excretion of catecholamines lasts for several days after surgery. Analysis of adrenal vein blood showed that either anaesthesia haemorrhage or tissue damage could stimulate adrenaline production.

Hypovolaemia is a strong stimulus for adrenomedullary activity and the restoration of blood volume reduces significantly previously induced secretion of catecholamines (Walker, 1959) (Fig. 22).

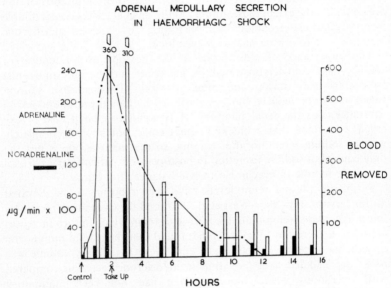

FIG. 22. Adrenal medullary secretion in haemorrhagic shock.

Experiments in animals have shown that the response to hypovolaemia does not occur if the adrenal glands have been denervated (Harrison, 1966). The afferent arc of this reflex pathway has not been identified. Other stimuli such as pain, fear, soft tissue injury can also produce a medullary response.

Interest has been focussed on the functional significance of the close proximity of the sources of catecholamines and cortisol. Anatomical studies have shown a rich vascular network between the cortex and the medulla, so that high concentrations of cortisol can enter the medulla and participate in the conversion of noradrenaline to adrenaline. Steroid administration in animals will produce an increased secretion of catecholamines by the adrenal medulla (Harrison, 1968).

There appears to be a synergistic relationship between cortisol and adrenaline secretion after trauma. It is suggested that the pressor effect of adrenaline in hypovolaemia is augmented by the simultaneous administration of cortisol but direct evidence is required to substantiate this. Adrenaline releases corticotrophin from the pituitary in both man and animals. Anaesthetic agents used in surgery have a variable effect on the adrenal medulla. Inhalation anaesthetics, such as ether, may stimulate secretion but in deep anaesthesia especially due to intravenous barbiturates the adrenal medullary secretion may be greatly diminished.

Relationships

The relationship between the adrenocortical and metabolic response to injury has been the subject of much speculation. Allbright (1943) observed a correlation between the excretion of potassium and nitrogen after injury and the increased function of the adrenal cortex. Moore and Ball (1952) drew attention to the similarity between the metabolic response and the effects of the administration of large doses of cortisone. It was then thought that the adrenocortical hormones initiated and controlled postoperative metabolic activity.

However, there is good evidence that all the postoperative metabolic changes cannot be explained in terms of altered adrenal function. Ingle (1951) introduced the concept of a permissive role for the adrenal in relation to metabolic activity after injury and suggested that adrenal secretions were necessary for metabolic activity, but that an increased output was not essential and that they did not cause the changes. Evidence for this permissive role came from both experimental and clinical studies. After major surgery the adrenal response is over long before the metabolic response. The response in patients undergoing adrenalectomy or hypophysectomy (and in those undergoing further surgery some time after these operations) follows a normal pattern so long as maintenance doses of cortisol are given during and after surgery. Constant replacement therapy does not, however, ensure a constant blood corticoid level after injury due to changes in hepatic conjugation and renal excretion, but large changes, similar to those recorded in intact subjects are unlikely to occur during constant dosage.

The administration of adrenocorticosteroids to nutritionally depleted animals will produce an increased excretion of nitrogen in the urine whereas a major operation in the presence of protein depletion has no effect on nitrogen excretion (Munro, 1966). Patients who are severely undernourished at the time of major surgery show a normal adrenocortical response.

Pancreatic Islets

Insulin

Hyperglycaemia occurs commonly soon after major injury and may persist for 2–3 days. The endocrine aspects of post-traumatic hyperglycaemia have been studied. Cortisol and adrenaline will stimulate gluconeogenesis and glycogenolysis and oppose the action of insulin (DeBodo and Altszuler, 1958) and both these substances are known to be increased after injury. Growth hormone is another insulin antagonist which appears in the serum in greater concentration immediately after injury.

The plasma insulin levels under resting conditions and at intervals after an infusion of glucose were measured before and after surgery using an immunoassay technique (Ross et al, 1966). The postoperative levels of insulin were found to be significantly higher than the pre-operative values at all times (Fig. 23). The increase was maximal on

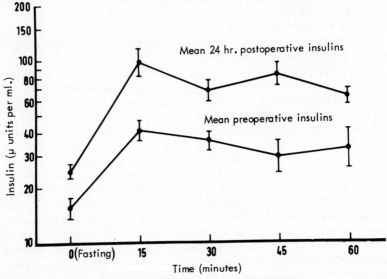

FIG. 23. Plasma insulin levels before and after operation. (Mean of six patients.)

the first postoperative day and normal levels were resumed in 3–4 days. An infusion of ACTH produced an increase in cortisol levels, and a reduction in glucose tolerance but had no effect on the level of circulating insulin. The alteration in carbohydrate metabolism appears to be due to the insulin antagonistic action of cortisol and perhaps also to some extent of growth hormone. Any explanation of the raised insulin levels after surgery must remain speculative and factors such as an impaired insulinase activity in the liver merit investigation. There is no information on the effect of injury on the secretion of insulin by the pancreas. Glucagon secretion after injury has not been determined.

Kidney

Erythropoeitin

This is a hormone which is thought to originate in the kidney and has the action of increasing the production of red blood cells in the bone marrow. Increased levels of erythropoeitin have been found in the plasma and the urine after haemorrhage.

Thyroid

Some aspects of the metabolic response to injury suggest the involvement of the thyroid. The rise in oxygen consumption, the oxidation of protein and fat are characteristic of overactivity by the thyroid. Accurate assessment of thyroid function has been difficult due to wide normal variations of most indices. The adrenal hormones which are available in excess amounts after trauma will also affect thyroid function.

Measurement of total protein bound iodine after operation as an index of total thyroxine in the plasma has shown an increase (Franksson et al, 1959), no change (Engstrom and Markarat, 1954) and even a reduction (Schwartz and Roberts, 1957).

The thyroid uptake of iodine is reduced after injury. This is a true reflection of the inability of the thyroid to handle iodine and is not a measure of the renal clearance of iodine (Johnston and Bell, 1965). The reduced uptake is also independent of other endocrine activity after trauma.

The peripheral metabolism of thyroxine can be assessed by measuring the urinary excretion of a tracer dose of ^{131}I thyroxine. Bernstein et al (1967) found an increase in the utilisation of thyroxine by the tissues in the first three days after surgery. Similar changes can be recorded when large doses of cortisone are given.

The most accurate measurement of thyroid function is the level of both thyroxine (T_4), Triiodothyronine (T_3) in bound and free forms in the plasma. These hormones are intimately bound to at least three proteins, thyroid binding globulin, albumin and pre-albumin of which albumin is the weakest carrier. A minute quantity of the total thyroxine (0.05%) exists in the free and unbound state in plasma. This fraction is able to enter the cell and influence intracellular metabolism. The level of free thyroxine is considered to be the true determinant of thyroid function with the protein bound hormone acting mainly as a large reservoir for free hormone. A reduction in the level of thyroid binding proteins produces an immediate rise in the concentration of free thyroxine.

The level of thyroid binding globulin is unchanged after surgery but the binding capacity of thyroid binding pre-albumin is reduced quickly after injury (Fig. 24) reaching its lowest level in the third day and and returning to normal in a week. Thyroid binding pre-albumin has a very short biological life of two days and the fall is probably due to an immediate reduction in anabolism of the protein after injury (Oppenheimer et al, 1965).

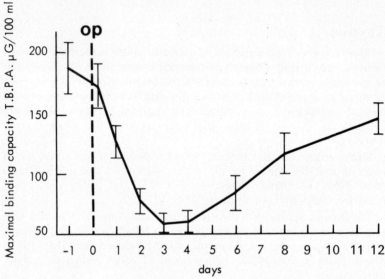

FIG. 24. Thyroid binding pre-albumin after operation.

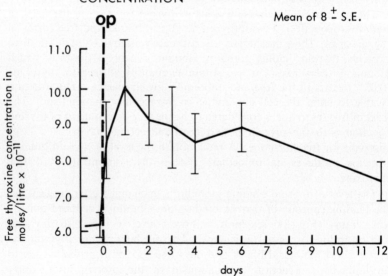

FIG. 25. Free thyroxine levels after surgery.

The level of free thyroxine (T_4) and Triiodothyronine (T_3) in plasma rises rapidly within a few hours of trauma (Fig. 25). The fall in binding protein may liberate more free hormone into the plasma. These alterations in the peripheral transport of thyroxine are occurring at a time when there is no measurable change in total thyroxine as measured by the protein bound iodine levels. The immunoassay of thyroid stimulating hormone in the blood also shows no increase after surgery (Kirby and Johnston 1970).

It would appear that the reduction in thyroid binding pre-albumin is a physiological regulatory mechanism, whereby the amount of thyroxine (T_4) available for cellular activity can be rapidly even though temporarily increased without any major change in total circulating hormone. A shift of thyroxine into cells after injury has important metabolic consequences such as an increase in the incorporation of amino acids into protein (Sokoloff, 1963). Protein for repair purposes is used extensively after trauma and the thyroid may be the initiating anabolic hormone of the injury period.

Activation of the Endocrine Response

Much has been written about the nature and extent of the endocrine response but much less is known with certainty about the mechanisms by which tissue damage initiates such a widespread response. The nervous system is of central importance (Fig. 19). Franksson and Gemzell (1955) demonstrated that psychic stimuli associated with the apprehension and fear attendant upon a surgical operation can cause the release of not only cortisol but also catecholamines and aldosterone. Drugs such as morphine and chlorpromazine used for premedication can stimulate the release of adrenocorticotrophic hormone, and fever, anaesthetic agents and bacterial toxins are other potent stimuli. The central nervous system is linked with the vascular tree by way of various volume and pressor receptors, and activation of these by acute blood loss stimulates the release of hormones which will in turn control the metabolism of minerals and water.

Hume and Egdahl (1960) have drawn attention to the importance of afferent sensory nerves by experiments in anaesthetised animals. Egdahl's model was an isolated limb preparation with only an artery, vein and sciatic nerve intact. Injury to the isolated limb produced an adrenocortical response only when the sciatic nerve was intact. Section of the spinal cord at C7 level also abolished the response. Pituitary stalk section did not affect the adrenal response to trauma, presumably due to ACTH releasing factors reaching the pituitary via routes other than the hypothalamohypophyseal portal system. Destruction of the anterior hypothalamus, leaving the pituitary gland intact completely abolished the response to injury. In man laparotomy is not followed by the normal adrenocortical reaction in the presence of a high spinal cord section; spinal anaesthesia on the other hand does not prevent a response to pelvic laparotomy although delaying its onset (Mattingly, 1967).

Some importance has been ascribed to so called "wound hormones" and agents such as histamine, 5-hydroxytryptamine and acetylcholine which are released in damaged tissue and thought to be capable of directly stimulating the adrenal. There seems little experimental evidence of a separate "wound hormone" as a method of stimulation.

The endocrine response is thus linked with many aspects of the metabolic response. Most of the endocrine effects have been found to be related quantitatively to the extent and severity of any injury or operation. Blood loss, tissue trauma and visceral stimuli are all components of many surgical situations which lead to direct contact with the central systems. Many of the stimuli arising during operation can be controlled by the maintenance of vascular homeostasis and the gentle handling of tissues, so that the first step in recovery begins with a skilful and gentle operative technique.

REFERENCES

Cooper, C. E. and Nelson, D. H. (1962). ACTH levels in plasma in pre-operative and surgically stressed patients. *J. Clin. Invest.* **41,** 1599.

Johnston, I. D. A. and Hadden, D. (1963). Effect of human growth hormone on postoperative nitrogen balance. *Lancet* **i,** 584.

Gemzell, C. A. (1962). Influence of growth hormone and nutrition in health and disease. Ciba Symposium on Protein Metabolism. Berlin.

Matsumoto, K., Takeyasu, K., Mizutani, S., Hamanaka, Y. and Vozumi, T. (1970). Plasma testosterone levels following surgical stress. *Acta Endocrinol.* **65,** 11.

Charters, A. C., Odell, W. D. and Thompson, J. C. (1969). Anterior pituitary function during surgical stress and convalescence. *J. Clin. Endocr.* **29,** 63.

Jones, C. M. and Eaton, F. B. (1933). Postoperative nutritional oedema. *Arch. Surg.* **27,** 659.

Coller, F. A., Fob, V., Vaughn, H. N., Kalder, N. B. and Moyer, C. A. (1945). Translocation of fluid produced by intravenous administration of fluids postoperatively. *Ann. Surg.* **122,** 663.

Cline, T. N., Cole, J. W. and Holden, W. D. (1953). Demonstration of an antidiuretic substance in the urine of postoperative patients. *Surg. Gynec. Obstet.* **96,** 674.

Moran, W. H., Miltenberger, F. W., Shuayb, W. A. and Zimmerman, B. (1964). The relationship of antidiuretic hormone secretion to surgical stress. *Surgery,* **56,** 99.

Verney, E. B. (1947). The antidiuretic hormone and the factors which determine its release. *Proc. roy. Soc. Lond.* **135,** 25.

Henry, J. P., Gauer, O. H. and Reeves, J. L. (1956). Evidence for atrial location of receptors influencing urine flow. *Circ. Res.* **4,** 85.

Cannon, W. B. (1929). Bodily changes in pain, hunger, fear and rage. Appleton & Co. New York.

Selye, H. (1946). General adaptation syndrome and diseases of adaptation. *J. clin. Endrocrinol.* **6**, 117.

Franksson, C. and Gemzell, C. A. (1954). Blood levels of 17 hydroxy-corticosteroids in surgery. *Acta chir. Scand.* **106**, 24.

Hume, D. M., Bell, C. C. and Barter, F. M. (1962). Direct measurement of adrenal secretion during operative trauma. *Surgery*, **52**, 174–186.

Gann, D. S. and Egdahl, R. H. (1965). Responses of adrenal corticosteroid secretion to hypotension and hypovolaemia. *S. Forum* **15**, 8.

Espiner, E. A. (1966). Urinary cortisol excretion in stress situations and in patients with Cushing's syndrome. *J. Endocrin*, **35**, 29.

Moore, F. D., Steenburg, R. W., Ball, M. R., Wilson, G. M. and Myrden, J. A. (1955). Studies in surgical endocrinology—The urinary excretion of 17 hydroxycorticosteroids in cases of soft tissue trauma. *Ann. Surg*, **141**, 145.

Tanaka, H., Manabe, H., Koshcyama, K., Hamaraka, Y., Matsumoto, K. and Uozumi, T. (1970). Excretion patterns of 17 ketosteroids and 17 hydroxycorticosteroids in surgical stress. *Acta Endocr*, **65**, 1–10.

Llaurado, J. G. (1955). Increased excretion of aldosterone immediately after operation. *Lancet* **i**, 1295.

Bartter, F. C., Liddle, G. W., Duncan, L. E., Barber, J. K. and Dilea, C. (1956). The regulation of aldosterone secretion in man—The role of fluid volume. *J. Clin. Invest*, **35**, 1306.

Skillman, J. J., Lauler, D. P., Hickler, R. B., Lyons, J. H., Olson, J. E., Ball, M. R. and Moore, F. D. (1967). Haemorrhage in man: Effect on renin, cortisol, aldosterone and urine composition. *Ann. Surg.* **166**, 865.

Kay, R. G. (1968). The effect of an aldosterone antagonist upon the electrolyte response to surgical trauma. *Brit. J. Surg*, **55**, 266.

Walker, W. F. (1965). Adrenal response to cardiac surgery. *Proc. roy. Soc. Med*, **58**, 1015.

Walker, W. F., Zileil, M. S., Reutter, F. W., Shoemaker, W. C. and Moore, F. D. (1959). Adrenomedullary secretion in haemorrhagic shock. *Amer. J. Physiol*, **197**, 773.

Harrison, T. S., Seaton, J. and Bartlett, J. Jnr. (1966). Adrenergic mechanisms in hypovolaemia. *Surg. Forum*, **17**, 66.

Harrison, T. S., Chawla, R. C. and Wojtalik, R. S. (1968). Steroidal influences on catecholamines. *New Engl. J. Med*, **279**, 136.

Albright, F. (1943). Relationship of Cushing's Syndrome to the reaction of the body to injurious agents. *Harvey Lect. Ser.* **38**, 123.

Ingle, D. J. (1954). The permissive action of hormones. *J. Endocr.* **14**, 1272.

Ross, H., Johnston, I. D. A., Welborn, T. A. and Wright, A. D. (1966). Effect of abdominal operation on glucose tolerance and serum levels of insulin, growth hormone and hydrocortisone. *Lancet* **ii**, 563.

Munro, H. N. (1966). Wound Healing (Sir Charles Illingworth). London. Churchill.

Franksson, C., Hastad, K. and Larsson, L. G. (1959). Effect of surgical stress on the hormonal release from the thyroid gland. *Acta chir. scand.* **264**, 118.

Engstrom, W. W. and Markardt, B. J. (1954). The serum precipitable iodine in surgical stress and serious illness. *J. clin. Invest.* **33**, 931.

Schwartz, A. E. and Roberts, K. E. (1957). Alterations in thyroid function following trauma. *Surgery* **42**, 814.

Johnston, I. D. A. and Bell, T. K. (1965). The effect of surgical operation on thyroid function. *Proc. roy. Soc. Med.* **58**, 1017.

Bernstein, G., Hasen, J. and Oppenheimer, J. H. (1967). The turnover of ^{131}I thyroxine in patients subjected to surgical trauma. *J. clin. Endocr.* **27**, 741.

Oppenheimer, J. H., Surks, M. I., Bernstein, G. and Smith, J. Crispin (1965). *Science* **149**, 748.

Kirby, R. and Johnston, I. D. A. (1971). The effect of operation on thyroid function. *Brit. J. Surg.* **58**, 303.

Sokoloff, L., Kaufman, S., Campbell, P. L., Francis, C. M. and Gelboin, H. V. (1963). Thyroxine stimulation of amino acid incorporation into protein. *J. Biol. Chem.* **238**, 1432.

Hume, D. M. and Egdahl, R. H. (1959). The importance of the brain in the endocrine response to injury. *Ann. Surg.* **150**, 697.

Johnston, I. D. A. (1968). The endocrine response to trauma. Scientific Basis of Medicine. Annual Reviews, p. 224.

Zimmermann, B. (1965). Pituitary and adrenal function in relation to surgery. *Surg. Clin. N. Amer.* **45**, 2, 299.

5: Circulatory Homeostasis

The past few years have seen a tremendous increase in our ability to study patients with disturbances of the cardiovascular system. This has been due, not to newer concepts in the causation of these disturbances, but to the availability of techniques for measurement of the various haemodynamic parameters, virtually at the bedside. Patient monitoring and intensive care units now abound and quantitative studies of patients in shock or severe distress are an essential feature of modern hospitals.

The basic physiology of the circulation is expressed clearly in numerous physiological text books. Our purpose here is to look at measurements actually made on patients with regard to the underlying physiological principles involved and their value in clinical practice.

1. Blood Volume

The methods of measuring total blood volume, plasma and red cell volume in clinical practice have already been mentioned. These measurements are valuable in experimental studies in animals and in steady state measurements in man. In most hospitals however they are neither readily available nor very accurate when needed most as in the patient in shock. It is easy to inject a known amount of I^{131} labelled albumin and wait 10–15 minutes before withdrawing the sample to allow calculation on the dilution principle already enunciated. Practically, however, we find that the albumin or the instrument may not be readily available and even if so, the equilibration time in the patient in shock is known to be prolonged so that the exact time when the sample should be removed is uncertain. Also our efforts are bent on resuscitation with intra-venous fluid replacement so that the steady state necessary for meaningful results is not usually possible.

Thus we come to rely on the assumed blood volume related to the individual weight. After resuscitation, when the patient's life is no longer in danger, a more reliable measurement of blood volume may be made, and the presence of over or under transfusion detected. It should be emphasised that one measurement of blood volume is of limited use. Of much better value are serial measurements showing a response to treatment.

2. *Haematocrit or Packed Cell Volume (P.C.V.)*

The venous Haematocrit is one of the commonest basic measurements made in blood analysis. Blood is collected from a vein without stasis into an anticoagulant. It is spun in a Wintrobe tube at 2500 r.p.m. for 30 minutes. The plasma and red cells separate off into different layers and the relationship or volume of one to the other and to the whole blood is read off. This is the large vessel haematocrit (L.V.H.) in contrast to the total body haematocrit (T.B.H.) which is the ratio or comparison of the measured red cell volume to the total blood volume and represents the whole circulation, whereas the L.V.H. represents that in the large vessels only. The difference between the two is said to be due to plasma skimming in the small vessels. The ratio of T.B.H./L.V.H. is normally about 0·92.

In clinical practice it is rare to measure the T.B.H. as the information gained of shift of red cells into or out of the micro-circulation may not be entirely accurate—an increased ratio is said to suggest a relative shift of red cells into the small vessels and vice versa.

Value of Haematocrit

Reflecting, as it does, the proportion of R.B.C.'s to total blood, it is raised if there is an increase in the R.B.C.'s or a fall in plasma volume.

L.V.H. → Increased ⎰ Excess R.B.C. e.g. Polycythaemia
⎱ Fall in Plasma Vol. e.g. Plasma loss. (Burns)

or

P.C.V. → Decreased ⎰ Excess Plasma e.g. Overhydration
⎱ Fall in R.B.C. e.g. anaemia, Blood loss.

FIG. 26. Changes in haematocrit (P.C.V.).

An example of the former is polycythaemia and of the latter plasma loss as in burns or peritonitis, or loss of the fluid and electrolyte constituents as in severe dehydration. A pure water loss does not change the haematocrit: a saline loss does produce a rise. The haematocrit fall is due to a fall in R.B.C. volume as in anaemia or blood loss or to an increase in plasma volume as in overhydration or overtransfusion with plasma. These changes are summarised in Fig. 26.

Many of the above factors may be present in a patient so that a change in haematocrit should be assessed carefully. After haemorrhage there is no immediate change as whole blood is lost. A few hours later when the impact of transcapillary migration of fluid is becoming manifest the L.V.H. will fall according to the degree of blood loss. After a few days the haematocrit is restored to normal by return of the R.B.C.'s to the blood from the bone marrow. This "pure" situation is seldom seen clinically as blood loss is treated by transfusion with low haematocrit blood or with plasma or plasma substitutes, which themselves alter the haematocrit. Also cells, which have been "trapped" in the micro-circulation, appear later in the circulation when the blood volume has been restored.

3. Cardiac Output

This is the output of blood from the heart per minute and can be measured in a number of ways, two of which will be mentioned.

(a) The Fick principle

This involves the analysis of blood samples taken from different parts of the circulation and measuring the oxygen uptake by the lungs:—

$$\text{Cardiac Output in L/min.} = \frac{\text{Oxygen consumption (ml/min.)}}{\text{Arterio-venous oxygen difference (ml/L)}}$$

Theoretically pulmonary artery blood should be removed to represent mixed venous blood. Usually a sample from a catheter in the right atrium is taken instead. Arterial blood is removed from a systemic artery. These samples are taken during collection of expired air to measure oxygen uptake. The accuracy of this method requires that the patient be in a steady state. It is therefore of doubtful value in patients in shock, but can be used in the study of cardiac conditions.

(b) Dye dilution technique

The cardiac output can be calculated from the concentration of a given dye as it passes a given point in the systemic circulation. Indocyanine green is injected through a central venous catheter and the time of injection is recorded electrically. Arterial blood is withdrawn by a constant withdrawal syringe and the blood passed through a densitometer. A dye curve is obtained and is recorded on a direct writing recorder. The problem now is the analysis of the curve. Previously planimetry was required but the computer has made for easier and speedier analysis. The problem of recirculation of the dye and extrapolation of the exponential decrease in dye concentration are dealt with by the computer. The normal cardiac output in a healthy young man is about 4 l/min. This is expressed usually in relation to the surface area of the body to allow ready comparison. The surface area of the average normal man is taken as 1·73 sq m.

$$\text{The cardiac index} = \frac{\text{Cardiac output}}{1 \cdot 73}$$

$$= 3 \cdot 12 \ 1/\text{min}/\text{m}^2$$

The stroke volume or output per ventricle is simply the cardiac output divided by the pulse rate. This is usually 60–120 ml/beat. For the corresponding stroke index, cardiac index is used instead of cardiac output.

Abnormal Cardiac Output

There is of course a tremendous reserve in the heart which can increase its output from 4 to 35 l/min. This is seen especially with severe exercise but some increase does occur with excitement, fear, cardiac disease, arteriovenous fistulae and diseases such as thyrotoxicosis. The contrast, diminished output, is seen with myocardial failure, cardiac abnormalities, severe anaemia, myxoedema and debilitating illness. Surgeons are primarily interested in changes in cardiac output following haemorrhage and shock.

Cournand et al (1943) found that the cardiac output decreased in shock while the peripheral resistance increased. Since then many studies have confirmed their results. In shock however there are difficulties in analysis. The low flow states have such a slow circulation time, and mixing is so disturbed, that measurements under these conditions are unlikely to be accurate. They probably however have relevance from a quantitative point of view. The whole problem of cardiac output is suitably reviewed physiologically by Guyton (1963) and in shock by Shoemaker (1967).

4. Cardiac Pressures

These are measured by cardiac catheterisation, at first only on the right side but later by trans-septal puncture also on the left side. The normal values are shown in Table 24. Their main value has been in the evaluation of cardiac problems but now they are increasingly being used in the study of circulatory homeostasis.

Table 24.

Cardiac Pressures

Right Atrium	−2 +5 mmHg
Right Ventricle	20 mmHg
Pulmonary Artery	20 mmHg
Left Atrium	20 mmHg
Left Ventricle	120 mmHg

The *right atrial pressure* (R.A.P.) is especially useful and is usually termed the central venous pressure (C.V.P.). A rise in the *right* ventricular pressure (R.V.P.) suggests a pulmonary artery stenosis or a septal defect. The pulmonary artery pressure may be raised from a high pulmonary blood flow due to septal defects or to pulmonary artery thickening or back-pressure from the left side of the heart as in mitral stenosis. The pulmonary blood flow can be calculated using the Fick principle taking samples from pulmonary artery and pulmonary vein (or allow oxygen saturation of 97% for this). From the pulmonary flow and pressure the pulmonary vascular resistance can be calculated:—

$$\frac{\text{Pulmonary Vascular Resistance}}{\text{mmHg/l/min}} = \frac{\text{mean pressure difference mmHg}}{\text{blood flow l/min}}$$

The *left atrial pressure* (L.A.P.) is only measurable by trans-septal catheterisation or at cardiac operation. This is unfortunate as it could be one of the most valuable parameters to measure. A rise in L.A.P is seen with mitral valve disease and a failing left ventricle. In the terminal stage of shock the L.A.P. rises as the cardiac output falls (Crowell and Guyton, 1961). The left ventricular pressure is similar to aortic pressure. It rises with obstructive valvular disease and increased peripheral resistance and decreased blood volume.

5. Peripheral Circulation

The terms macro-circulation and micro-circulation are in common use. Their main value has been to create some interest in the distal part of the circulatory system which has to some extent been neglected in favour of the heart and major vessels.

The micro-circulation is defined here as that part of the circulation between the arterioles and venules. Its importance is reflected by the fact that it contains a major part of the blood volume; that its tone and capacity reflects the peripheral resistance; that within it the blood to tissue cell exchanges take place and finally that by fluid shift it controls blood volume. In brief it controls blood pressure, nutrient exchange and blood volume.

It is wise however to consider the circulation in continuity when investigating disease and planning rational therapy.

As blood passes from the heart down the major vessels the flow is pulsatile and the pressure is high (Fig. 27). When it enters the smaller vessels, e.g. muscular arteries, the amplitude of pulsation becomes smaller and the pressure gradually falls. This is progressive as the calibre of the vessels diminish, until in the arterioles the flow is even and the pressure down to about one third of systolic. These vessels are extremely important in providing the main peripheral resistance to the flow of blood by their number and by the tone in their muscular walls. The tone governs the radius of the vessels and through Poiseuille's law the flow, which is further controlled by the precapillary sphincter. Flow and pressure in the capillary system is controlled by the two sphincters pre and post capillary so that the blood passing into the venules has a very low pressure. The venous side of the circulation is also very important especially as a capacitance compartment. Despite the low mean pressure of about 7 cm of water they accommodate a large fraction of the blood volume because they are easily distensible. Indeed Gauer and Henry (1963) regarded this as a key factor in the regulation of normal blood volume and in the rapid changes of cardiac output. The capacitance value is easily demonstrated clinically by observing the benefit in raising the foot of the bed in shock patients.

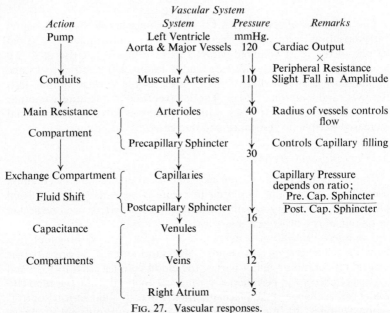

FIG. 27. Vascular responses.
Factors related to changes in pressure within the vascular system.

The microcirculation is under the control of neural, hormonal, and locally produced substances. The neural control is largely vaso-constrictive; the metabolic factors vasodilatory. The more distal parts of the system are more under the control of locally produced metabolites than under neural control. As the vessels get smaller the physical properties of the blood become more important, notably the size and number of erythrocytes and the size of other molecules in the plasma; factors responsible for the viscosity of the blood—a complex and still not completely understood subject. The viscosity of the blood is related almost exponentially to the haematocrit. It is influenced also by the high molecular weight proteins especially fibrinogen and by any abnormal proteins present. Aggregation of R.B.C.'s which occur in low flow states will increase viscosity as also will a fall in pH. Presumably any increase in viscosity occurring in association with a low flow state will have a particularly bad effect in the venules where stagnation is common and thrombosis an obvious hazard. This knowledge has led to therapeutic attempts to keep the viscosity low by infusion of crystalloids or low molecular weight dextran in the hope of improving flow through the microcirculation. A haematocrit value of about 30% is probably best as it allows maximum oxygen transport capacity combined with maximum flow through the tissues.

Assessment of Peripheral Circulation

(a) Clinical Features

The first assessment is obviously a clinical one, when the colour and temperature of the skin of the limbs, the colour of the fingernails, and the response of skin and nails to pressure is observed. The state of venous filling when the patient is horizontal is also important. All this should be observed in conjunction with the general colour of the patient especially the face and conjunctiva, his demeanour, the respiratory rate, pulse, etc.

A normal peripheral circulation is characterised by a pink warm skin with pink toe nails and quick return to normal after blanching by finger pressure. The veins should be visible and well filled. Empty veins which do not fill up after stroking them proximally suggest that hypovolaemia is present.

The blue cold skin of peripheral circulatory failure is due to extreme arteriolar vasconstriction with stagnation of the blood in the capillaries and venules from lack of vis-a-tergo.

The pulse rate in circulatory failure is usually rapid and of poor quality. But a slow pulse may be present especially where myocardial failure is present also. Further measurements are required to evaluate the circulatory status of the patient.

(b) Blood Pressure

Blood pressure is usually measured by auscultation using a sphygmomanometer. In intensive care units, recovery units or in an emergency situation an arterial catheter may be preferred. This can be introduced into the femoral artery percutaneously or by cut down into the radial artery if necessary. The catheter is connected via a transducer to a recorder. The catheter requires to be filled with heparinised saline to prevent clotting. It is however the most accurate way of continual assessment of blood pressure. Various appliances have been devised to obviate arterial catheterisation. They are satisfactory at near normal pressures but their value drops off as the pressure falls.

Clinicians sometimes become overconcerned with the systolic blood pressure, which can be misleading. We must remember that when the circulatory system is stressed compensatory mechanisms come into play to maintain the blood pressure at normal levels. Thus a normal blood pressure gives no indication that something may be wrong which requires treatment before collapse occurs. The compensatory mechanisms involved are arteriolar constriction with a rise in peripheral resistance and increases in cardiac output.

A raised peripheral resistance can be detected by pallor of the skin, coldness, slow refilling and a rise in the diastolic blood pressure which results in a pulse low in volume.

Increased cardiac output is due to increased cardiac rate. A fall in the systolic blood pressure means that the circulatory compensatory mechanisms have been swamped. The vasoconstriction occurs mainly in the skin and in some organs. It is not uniform so that blood flow to various organs is different (Catchpole et al, 1953).

(c) Central Venous Pressure

This might more appropriately be considered with cardiac haemo-dynamics but, as it is such a common measurement in the shock patient, and is used in conjunction with other parameters of the peripheral circulation, it is dealt with here.

It is measured by a catheter inserted into the basilic vein and passed up into the superior vena cava or better the right atrium. The catheter is connected by a Y tube to a long plastic tube which is fastened to a vertical centimetres scale. The zero is marked level with the mid-thoracic region—the level of the right atrium. This is obviously a somewhat rough approximation so that the final figures must be considered in the same way. The other limb of the Y is connected to a saline bottle and the catheter is kept open by a slow infusion.

When a pressure reading is required the catheter is clipped off, the measuring tube filled with saline from the bottle and the bottle is now clipped off and the catheter clip removed. Saline will flow into the catheter until the pressure is stabilised and can be read off the vertical scale in cms of saline (mmHg).

The normal C.V.P. is approximately 5 cms saline. It varies with respiration so that on deep inspiration a normal pressure is -2 cm saline. For practical clinical purposes the positive value of about $+5$cm is accepted as being the normal one.

The C.V.P. is influenced by the blood volume being low in hypo-volaemia. A figure of more than 10 cms saline would suggest over-transfusion. The C.V.P. is also however, influenced by the state of the heart and rises with congestive cardiac failure. It is thus a balance between blood returning to the heart and the heart's ability to expel it. It is a mistake to think of C.V.P. as being synonymous with the total blood volume. Indeed where the two have been measured simultaneously and correlated it was found that the blood volume needed to be 40% above the predicted normal to maintain a normal C.V.P. (Prout,

1968). It should therefore be equated with effective circulating blood volume. If the C.V.P. is maintained at the upper limit of normal (+10 cm saline), then any circulatory inefficiency present could not be due to inadequate blood volume and more blood should not therefore be needed (McGowan and Walters, 1965).

(d) Peripheral Resistance

This as already mentioned is the resistance to the flow of blood through the distal vessels particularly the arterioles. It cannot be measured directly and must therefore be calculated from a formula.

$$\text{Total peripheral resistance (T.P.R.)} = \frac{\text{Mean arterial pressure} - \text{C.V.P. mmHg}}{\text{cardiac index L/min/m}^2}$$

$$\text{Normal} = 29 \cdot 0 \pm 1 \cdot 0 \text{ units}$$

The mean arterial pressure (M.A.P.) is a systolic and diastolic mean of the arterial blood pressure taken from a pressure recorder and is usually about 95 mmHg.

Although at present peripheral resistance is rarely calculated it is likely that in further studies, where the controversy of vasoconstrictor versus vasodilator drugs is being explored, it will be calculated more often. A high peripheral resistance is shown clinically by a cold pale skin. A low resistance by a warm dry skin. Which is most advantageous in a given situation is still sub judice.

6. Abnormal Situations

1. Haemorrhage

The physiological reaction to bleeding has to some extent been dealt with previously. Haemorrhage produces a response of the defence mechanisms in the body, commensurate with its severity and circulatory, nervous, hormonal and renal mechanisms are called into play (Fig. 28). Volume and pressure receptors in the atria, aortic and carotid areas are stimulated. The arterioles and precapillary sphincters contract and the venous tone increases to accommodate for the diminished blood volume. The nervous reaction is assisted or backed up by a hormonal one in which the adrenal plays the major part. Catecholamines, principally adrenaline but also noradrenaline, are released in proportion to the degree of bleeding. This increased excretion is returned to normal by re-infusion of shed blood (Walker et al, 1959). The same is true for adrenal cortical secretion of 17 Hydroxy-Corticosteroids (Hume and Nelson, 1954, Walker et al, 1959).

The catecholamines are vasoconstrictors and their action is said to be supported by the steroids. However in large doses the steroids reduce the peripheral resistance (Dietzman and Lillehei, 1969). Increased release of pitressin (A.D.H.) associated with reduced blood volume results in oliguria and stimulation of the renin/angiotensin system brings about release of aldosterone and retention of sodium. The renal mechanism controls blood volume by diminishing loss of water in the urine and by maintaining osmotic pressure by sodium retention. The neuro-hormonal influence sustains the existing blood volume to keep it efficient. Meanwhile, in the capillaries the fluid exchange serves to increase the blood volume by transporting water from the tissues into the vascular system. The later replenishment of plasma proteins and red cells has already been stated.

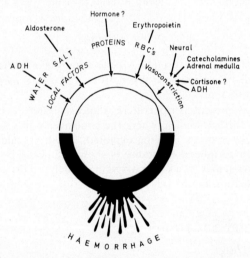

Fig. 28. Compensatory mechanisms in shock.

Treatment

For loss of blood the only true therapy is to replace blood. If the loss is not severe the body's compensatory mechanisms will be sufficient. But if blood pressure falls then blood is needed. Until this is available blood substitutes may be given.

2. Shock

This is a difficult term to define, and, being so, to describe as a definite entity. The boundary between normality and the state we call shock is a wide one, which cross unknowingly because the blood pressure is normal and indeed can be raised, the pulse rate is regular and slow, and clinical signs are not self-evident. It is this boundary zone that is really interesting since a warning of impending shock could result in timely treatment. We must accept therefore two stages in circulatory inadequacy, a pre-shock subclinical stage and a stage of clinical shock. Once this is accepted definition becomes easier. The pre-shock stage is one where circulatory inadequacy has led to poor tissue perfusion with damage to tissue cells, which later beomes manifest clinically as a collapsed patient with hypotension.

Anoxia of the tissue cells leads to damage to the mitochondria and depressed formation of high energy phosphate bonds. Diminution of energy means inadequate cell metabolism with release of organic acids which can produce acidosis, and enzymes which may play a part in producing further trouble. An increase in the Kinins, Kallikrein and other substances in the circulation can produce deleterious effects on capillaries, further aggravating the state of hypotension.

The changes produced in the cardiovascular system have already been alluded to in discussing the effects of haemorrhage. Further to these is the sludging of red cells in the microcirculation especially in the post-capillary venules throughout the body and in the sinusoids of the liver (Shoemaker, 1967). This aggregation of cells withdraws them from the general circulation and depresses further the effective blood volume. It accounts for the "sequestration" of red cells which may, on recovery, re-enter the circulation. A further effect of this pheno-menon is to increase the viscosity of the blood and slow down even more the blood flow through the capillaries. Anoxia, metabolic acidosis, low flow, aggregation of cells, increased viscosity liberation of local metabolites all act to produce deterioration in the situation and produce a vicious cycle while the arterioles and precapillary sphincters are partially closed to sustain peripheral resistance while the rest of the microcirculation is undergoing vasodilation from local metabolites, etc. A point may be reached in the shock state when this arteriolar vaso-constriction is present at the expense of the body, i.e. a mechanism which was at first life-saving is now in danger of destroying life. Thus the concept of releasing the vasoconstriction by drugs was developed principally by Nickerson (1955). The problem is when and when not to interfere therapeutically.

Effect of Shock on Organs

The variable response of the different vascular beds to the stimulus of increased sympathetic activity results in differential perfusion of various tissues in the body. This and other factors can affect organ function to the detriment of the patient. A few salient points deserve further mention.

Heart. A fall in cardiac output is known to occur in shock especially due to hypovolaemia. It has unfortunately been assumed that there is always a low cardiac output in shock. Studies have have shown this to be untrue, especially in traumatic shock (Shoemaker, 1967,

Shoemaker, and Walker, 1969), and in septic shock (Cohn et al, 1967) when a high cardiac output is often present. The value of this high output is lost by shunting through arteriovenous anastomoses (Duff et al, 1969).

Kidney. A fall in renal blood flow is an invariable accompaniment of shock and is due to sympathetic constrictor activity as well as low blood volume. The oliguria which results is usually temporary but if sepsis is present or pigments accumulate in the blood, renal failure may occur.

Lungs. Blaisdell et al (1970) reviewed the changes in the lungs in patients who had died in shock. They included atelectasis, pulmonary congestion going on to intra-alveolar haemorrhages, and pulmonary oedema. Pulmonary thromboembolism may occur and lead on to microvascular obstruction with damage to the alveolar and endothelial cells. This and the release of substances which produce broncho and venoconstriction can severely affect the ventilation perfusion of the lung, reduce the arterial Po_2 and eventually lead to complete ventilatory failure.

Liver. Early on in the shock state there is an increased hepatic blood flow and later increased hepatic resistance. This, if prolonged, may affect the metabolism of the liver and also contribute to the sequestration of blood in the splanchnic area (Shoemaker, 1967).

Causes of Shock

Virtually any condition which can affect the circulatory system can produce shock. Broadly speaking shock can be divided into two main types. 1. Oligaemic shock. 2. Normovolaemic shock.

(a) Oligaemic Shock

This is by far the commonest group. The basic underlying cause is a fall in blood volume which can be due to loss of whole blood, plasma, red cells, water and salts. The loss may be internal and therefore not easily appreciated or external and self-evident. Also self-evident is the treatment which is simply to replace what is lost. It would be tempting to say replace volume for volume, but studies in injured soldiers with severe shock have shown that more than the amount lost must be replaced. Indeed an excess blood volume may be required to sustain life. In every case a central venous catheter should be inserted and extreme care exercised when the venous pressure rises to $+10$ cm saline.

The work of Shires et al (1961) on the losses of "functional" extra-cellular fluid after operation led to the use of Ringer lactate in quite large amounts as well as blood. It could be given during any major operation but especially during surgery in a shocked patient (Shires, 1967, Crocker, 1968, Dudley et al, 1968). This approach is still, we believe, sub judice and should only be used by those prepared to be most meticulous in their care and monitoring of patients. The danger, of pulmonary oedema, is a very real one and should make most of us rely on replacing what is lost. Extra sodium bicarbonate may be of value if acidosis is present or expected.

(b) Normovolaemic Shock

This has many causes which have this in common that they do not produce loss of blood volume. Certainly the "effective" blood volume is diminished by pooling of the blood in the blood vessels as in septic or endotoxic shock. Various causes will be discussed briefly.

(c) Cardiac Failure

In this the pump fails to sustain cardiac output. The treatment of this is discussed on p. 149.

(d) Neurogenic Shock

Shock was once thought to be related to severe pain but this must be very uncommon. Indeed severe pain was not obvious in many soldiers with ghastly injuries.

Perhaps a more common form of neurogenic shock is that seen after pulmonary embolus where partial occlusion only has occurred. There is thought to be associated spasm of the pulmonary artery, due to stimulation of autonomic receptors producing a state of shock out of proportion to the haemodynamic disturbance (Aviado and Schmidt, 1955). Another cause of neurogenic shock is injury to the spinal cord with tetraplegia which produces loss of vasoconstriction tone on the vessels and pooling of blood.

(e) Adrenal Failure

In patients with Addison's disease, the Friederichsen-Waterhouse syndrome, or those on long-term steroids who have surgery without steroid cover, shock may occur. It is relieved by giving hydrocortisone. At times adrenal failure is implicated in patients with haemorrhage or traumatic shock and who are refractory to therapy. This is a refuge of the destitute. Adrenal failure as a result of shock must be extremely rare. As an entity it has not been supported by animal studies (Walker et al, 1959b). This subject is discussed in Chapter 14.

(f) Septic Shock

This is probably the commonest cause of normovolaemic shock other than cardiac failure. It is certainly one which the surgeon must constantly bear in mind especially in elderly patients after prostatectomy or even urethral dilatation and those with gallbladder disease. The commonest type of septic shock accounting for nearly two-thirds of cases is endotoxic shock due to toxins released by gram negative bacteria, e.g. E. Coli. The toxins are said to stimulate the adrenal medulla and sympathetic nervous system with resulting arteriolar and venular vasoconstriction. Acidosis develops as a result of low tissue blood flow and this produces arteriolar dilatation. As the post capillary venules remain constricted, blood pools in the capillaries (Dietzman and Lillehei, 1968). The other cause of septic shock is that due to infection by gram positive organisms and accounts for perhaps one-third of the cases.

The main problem is one of diagnosis. One should suspect its possibility in any unexplained shock condition, especially in the type of patient already mentioned. The temperature may not be raised. Blood culture will support the diagnosis but in retrospect. The aspiration of pus from the chest or subphrenic space or its appearance in a catheter will also support the diagnosis. On many occasions however the diagnosis is treated first and proved later. An example may serve to emphasise this.

Case Report

A 74 year old man underwent prostatectomy. A very large prostate was removed and blood transfusion was given. About 6 days later he had a slight shivering spell and the temperature rose to 99·6°F. This passed off but 8 hours later he became unconscious with cold clammy pale skin with a tinge of blueness in it. His pulse was 150+/min. His systolic blood pressure was 65–70 mm of Hg. The catheter was changed. When the new one was put in some pus came out. He was treated with intravenous saline, antibiotics and nor-adrenaline. Next morning he was sitting up in bed reading a newspaper.

This patient emphasises the rapid onset and progression of the condition as well as the ready response to treatment. The use of a vasoconstrictor here seems at first illogical then logical if vasodilation is present. These will be discussed under therapy.

(g) Irreversible Shock

This is given a separate place in discussion not because it merits it as a separate, distinct entity, but because it is a dangerous term which may lull the doctor into a sense of "everything has been done, but. . .". A better term is that of refractory hypotension (Smith and Moore, 1962). In a careful study of 15 patients, classified as such, they described four groups.

1. With unrecognised volume deficits with hyponatraemia ± acidosis.
2. With severe shock.
3. With myocardial failure.
4. With local vascular complications of extensive operations.

The two commonest biochemical changes were hyponatraemia and metabolic acidosis. In 3 patients who died there was an adequate explanation at postmortem.

A further possibly overlooked cause of shock is disseminated intravascular coagulation (Hardaway, 1965). As its name suggests there is diffuse coagulation of the blood with a profound fall in the haemoglobin and in fibrinogen. The diagnosis rests on evidence of fibrinogen utilisation. If present heparin is required and possibly also blood transfusion.

(h) *Management of the Patient in Shock*

In an emergency situation such as this it is always comforting and clinically advantageous to have a system for tackling the problem. Let us suppose therefore that we are called to a patient in shock and the nurses are preparing for intravenous therapy. The history is either known or should be divulged during the initial period of observation and examination.

Taken step by by step we may proceed thus:—

1. Observe: Colour of face, conjunctiva and periphery.
            Respirations—must have adequate airway.
            Mental state—subdued, irrational, coma.
            Area of injury—for blood loss, compound fractures, etc.

2. Examination: Pulse rate, blood pressure, temperature of skin.
            State of veins especially on dorsum of foot.
            Recirculation after pressure.
            Source of bleeding. Signs of fractures.

Note: All the above is done very rapidly and if necessarily cursorily. Detailed examination must await resuscitation. But a quick examination can allow a rapid assessment of problem.

3. Take blood for cross matching, acid base parameters and electrolytes. Start I.V. fluids, either plasma expander or Group O blood if required, until cross-matched blood available.

4. Set up a central venous pressure line.

5. Even with a blood transfusion running at a fast rate so that drops have merged to a flow to give adequate replacement, the measurement of blood volume by R.I.S.A. etc. can begin.

6. Insert a Foley catheter and measure the hourly urine output.

7. A more detailed assessment of the cause of the shock can now take place. Fractures should be splinted and the patient prepared for operative treatment if necessary.

8. Consider E.C.G. blood culture, X-rays of chest, abdomen and limbs. Blood analysis for clotting factors, etc.

(*i*) Treatment of Shock

This obviously depends on the cause. That due to a specific organ e.g. the heart, will be discussed later. We will look mainly at hypovolaemic and septic shock as they are commoner in surgical cases. Blood transfusion is the mainstay of treatment with pharmacological agents a second best (except in septic shock).

1. Blood Transfusion

The problems in this relate to correct cross-matching, the amount required, the speed of infusion and the risks inherent in the use of blood.

Amount required

This depends on the severity of the shock and the response to treatment. The severity of shock can be estimated roughly from clinical signs and blood pressure as in Table 25. Fractures of long

Table 25.

Estimation of Degree of Shock

Degree	Systolic Blood Pressure	Loss of Blood Volume	Clinical Features
	mmHg		
Mild	90–100	20–25%	Anxiety, weakness, thirst, pulse 100 ↑
Moderate	70–90	30–35%	Restless, pale, greyskin, slow refilling of blanched skin pulse 120 ↑
Severe	< 70	40–50%	Comatose, mottled cyanotic skin, air-hunger pulse 140 ↑

N.B.   Small fall in blood pressure in previously **HYPERTENSIVE** patients may be *very* significant.

bones need one unit of blood per fracture. If more than two long bones are damaged or if the fracture is compound add a further 2 units. Pelvic fractures are notoriously "blood thirsty", and 2–3 units should be allowed for these. The total blood volume should be estimated from the body weight or from actual measurement and the amount of blood required calculated. As already mentioned volume for volume replacement may not be enough. Fortunately we have some parameters which help.

1. Skin should be warm, dry, pink with good filling veins.

2. C.V.P. should be 5 cms saline—no more than 10 cms saline.

3. Urine output—should be 40–60 ml/hour in the adult. Less in the child.

In burns a good guide is the percentage or area of the body surface burned.

To estimate this the rule of nines is helpful.

i.e. *Upper limbs*   9% body surface each   = 18%
    Lower limbs   Thigh, 9% body surface each = 18%
                 Below knee, 9% surface each = 18%
    Trunk   Front—18%   = 18%
                 Back—18%   = 18%
    Head and neck   = 9%
               Perineum   = 1%

As a rough measure the severity of shock in terms of blood loss in burns is approximately equivalent to the percentage burned (Shoemaker, 1967), e.g. 30% burn comparable to shock from loss of 30% of blood volume.

In treating shock from burns plasma rather than blood is required. But usually about one-third of the volume needs are made up by blood, two-thirds by plasma. More blood may be needed in large burns where significant haemolysis with haemoglobinuria may occur.

Rate of Infusion

This is governed by the response as above. The C.V.P. should be the guide to too rapid replacement. With a low C.V.P. the blood can be given very rapidly. In severe shock this may mean 500 ml of blood every 10 minutes until the C.V.P. starts to rise.

Risks inherent in use of blood

The main one which is usually avoided is mismatched transfusion. If sufficient time is given for cross-matching this should be negligible. In the meanwhile plasma or plasma substitute may be used. Over-transfusion is avoided by use of a C.V.P. line. Reactions of a minor and unspecified nature may arise. Hepatitis is a problem which is difficult to eradicate except by screening donors. Blood substitutes will be discussed later.

2. General Measures in Shock Therapy

The patient should be kept in a warm but not overheated bed. Elevation of the foot of the bed by about 15° helps to promote venous return. Nasogastric suction keeps the abdomen from becoming distended and lessens the risk of inhalation of vomitus. A pulse, blood pressure and vital signs chart is essential to ensure adequate supervision at all times. It may be necessary to turn the patient in prolonged intensive therapy to prevent bedsores. Special care should be taken with regard to the heart, lungs and kidneys.

Pharmacology of Shock
1. Vasoconstrictors versus Vasodilators

Vasoconstrictors (Noradrenaline, Aramine, Vasoxine) act by constricting the arterioles and venules of the skin, kidneys and splanchnic organs.   Arteriolar constriction raises the peripheral resistance and thence the blood pressure. Venular constriction aids in the return of blood to the heart. This, however, may be at the expense of blood flow through the tissues. There appears to be a critical point at which the rise in blood pressure is insufficient to push more blood through the narrowed vessels. The value of Vasoconstrictor drugs is in shock due to vasodilatation, i.e. in septic shock, after drugs such as chlorpromazine, and in neurogenic shock and anaesthesia. They have no beneficial effect in hypovolaemic shock and should not be used.

Vasodilators such as the alpha blocker phenoxybenzamine (Dibenzyline) or the beta stimulator isoproterenol (Isuprel) have the opposing action of relieving "excessive" vasoconstriction so that blood can flow through the tissues and abolishing tissue anoxia and acidosis.   The initiator of this method of treatment was Nickerson (1955) but many others have utilised it successfully. Vasodilatation will, however, drop the "effective circulating blood volume" and if this is low anyway a profound drop in blood pressure will occur with a deterioration in the clinical state.   Such therapy must be covered by C.V.P.   A plan of action might be:—

Measure C.V.P. and if it is low give a blood transfusion until the C.V.P. rises to 10 cm of saline. If the patient is still clinically vasoconstricted (pale, cold, clammy skin), then digitalis should be given to improve the cardiac action in case the high C.V.P. is due to this. If not improved and the measured blood volume is normal with a high C.V.P. vasodilatation should be produced by phenoxybenzamine 1 mg/Kg I.V. over a period of 4 hours. With this the blood pressure may fall a little, the C.V.P. should fall and the skin should become warm and pink. Another drug used is Isoproterenol in the dose of 0·02 ml/Kg/hour intravenously. The best situation for this is a high C.V.P. and a relatively slow pulse, i.e. about 80/100 min. Isuprel has both a chronotropic and inotropic action on the heart. It may produce extrasystoles at first and then fibrillation.   Its action should thus be observed by an E.C.G. When the heart speeds up the drug should be stopped immediately.

The temperature of the skin has also been used as a guide to vasodilator therapy. Recently Ross et al (1969) endorsed Ibsen's (1967) dictum—"open up and fill up—stop when the feet get warm". The rectal, skin, and big toe temperatures were measured. Divergence between the toe and rectal temperatures suggested hypovolaemia which might not be indicated by the C.V.P.—although usually it is. A variety of vasodilators were used, but always with careful monitoring of pulse rate, systemic blood pressure and C.V.P. which would fall, and would be raised to normal or to an acceptable level by giving blood rapidly. A good result would be matched by a return of skin temperature to normal—approximating the rectal temperature. Chlorpromazine (Largactil) 5 mgm was given intravenously and found to be a short-lasting vasodilator which did not produce a severe fall in systemic blood pressure. Phentolamine (Rogitine) was also used on occasion in doses of 2·5–10 mg intravenously and recently thymoxamine (Opilon) in doses of 0·1 mg/Kg body weight has been given. The shorter acting vasodilators were preferred to the longer acting phenoxy-benzamine. This use of skin and rectal temperature would seem to be a valuable adjunct to present means of guiding therapy and preventing "irreversible shock".

2. Hydrocortisone

This is given in varying doses according to guesswork as there is practically always enough endogenous cortisone present with the exception of high risk cases, i.e. patients already on cortisone. It is usually given in a dose of 100 mg intravenously and is said to augment the effect of endogenous catecholamines on blood vessels and yet in larger doses 50–100 mg/Kg it is used as a vasodilator agent which lowers the peripheral resistance by an unknown action. It is also said to have a beneficial effect on endotoxin shock provided that the correct antibiotic is used with it (Lillehei et al, 1964). If hydrocortisone is used, it is best not to expect too much from it.

3. Digitalis

This of course is used in shock associated with cardiac failure, and is therefore useful in the child with congenital heart disease or in the elderly patient. It undoubtedly has a place in therapy but is no panacea.

4. Antibiotics

These have been mentioned in the treatment of septic shock. What is the correct one or combination to be used? This largely depends on the organism involved and in the sensitivities formed to it locally. Gram positive organisms are responsible for roughly one-third of cases and gram negative organisms for the remaining two-thirds. The former are usually seen when the skin, subcutaneous tissues, bones and joints, lungs or heart are involved. Gram negative infections are common in abdominal surgery. Murdoch and his colleagues (1968) who have created such interest in the condition advise Kanamycin Sulphate as the first choice, when gram negative infection is suspected, in the dose of 250 mg six-hourly intramuscularly (in adults). Gentamycin is recommended against Pseudomonas pyocyaneus, E. Coli and Staph. aureus. Another wide spectrum antibiotic is Cephaloridine which has the advantage of being less toxic, but is not effective against Ps Pyocyaneus. Various combinations of the above may be used such as ampicillin and Cloxacillin or Kanamycin and Cloxacillin, with realisation of possible toxic effects. Problems of toxicity are relatively unimportant as the situation is usually life threatening.

5. Alkalis

In the treatment of acidosis Sodium Bicarbonate is normally used. Even before the results of acid base parameters are known it is customary to give 50 mEq of $NaHCO_3$ over about 20–30 minutes in anticipation of the acidosis. Sodium Lactate (M/6) has a similar but slightly slower effect.

Tris buffer and THAM used in open heart surgery is also an effective way of combating the acidosis of shock. A dose of 36 g in a litre of solution may be given over a two hour period (Shoemaker, 1968).

6. Mannitol

This is used to promote diuresis and eliminate the problem of renal failure in shock cases especially after crush injury. One hundred ml of a 20% solution may be infused over 30 minutes. If the urine output does not rise it can be repeated in 6 hours.

7. Crystalloids

The value of saline in shock has been known for 40 years, but was largely replaced by blood and blood substitutes as they become more readily available. Normal saline passes quickly from the vascular component into the rest of the E.C.F. It is still of use in making up for losses as in dehydration. More recently Brooks et al (1963) suggested the use of hypertonic saline to improve the osmolality of the E.C.F. as hypo-osmolality was seen in hypovolaemia. As regards this the present position is one of caution in its use as overloading with salt is possible. The use of Ringer lactate has already been mentioned. Another solution—Hartmanns has been advocated to make up for depletion of the E.C.F. This followed on the work of Shires et al (1964) who demonstrated the contraction of the E.C.F. after trauma. Doubts on the accuracy of E.C.F. measurements in non-steady states was expressed by MacLean (1968) among others. A reasonable balanced judgment would be that Hartmann's solution could be given in amounts up to 1–2 litres until blood was cross-matched (Eiseman 1967, Hardaway et al, 1967).

8. Blood Substitutes

There is no solution which has all the properties of blood. Thus there is no ideal blood substitute. A number of solutions have the power to expand the intravascular volume so maintaining the blood volume. These are useful when blood is not available, or when one is waiting for cross-matching, or in the treatment of mass casualties as in war (Walker, 1968). An excellent detailed analysis of blood replacement has been provided by Gruber (1969).

(a) Plasma

This is more ideal than whole blood in conditions where plasma loss predominates, e.g. burns and peritonitis or where the haematocrit is raised, e.g. dehydration present. The main problem is the risk of serum hepatitis. In Britain dried plasma is most commonly used because it is easily stored and is bacteriologically sterile. The risk of hepatitis is present, even as high as that for whole blood, roughly 10%; more if large amounts are used in a single patient.

In the U.S.A. the risk of hepatitis has been minimised by pooled plasma stored in liquid state at room temperature for 6 months. This has the disadvantage of storage problems and the risk of bacterial growth.

(b) Pasteurised Plasma Protein Solution—PP.S.

In this the virus of hepatitis is destroyed by pasteurisation. Its present main disadvantage is increased cost of production. But the elimination of virus hepatitis will probably encourage greater use of this solution in the future.

(c) Serum Albumin

This like the above is pasteurised to destroy the virus. It is supplied in bottles of 70 ml (25 gram) amounts, and again the cost is the main disadvantage.

(d) Dextrans

These are polysaccharides built up from glucose molecules. Two are in common use at present.

DEXTRAN High molecular weight (70,000+)

In view of its average molecular weight it is sometimes known as Dextran 70 (Macrodex:Dextraven). It is supplied as a 6% solution with or without saline and has the property of remaining in the vascular compartment for a considerable time, thus supporting the circulating volume. About 30% of the infused Dextran is excreted in the urine in 6 hours and about 40% in 24 hours. Usually not more than 1 litre is infused at any time as there is a risk of bleeding disorder with high dosage. It is valuable as an inexpensive, readily available, non toxic plasma expander. Blood for cross-matching should be removed before giving it because of the tendency for rouleaux formation.

Low molecular weight DEXTRAN (40,000)

This is usually known as Dextran 40 or according to the firms that supply it (Rheomacrodex:Lomodex). It is supplied as a 10% solution in saline or 5% dextrose. About 60% of the infused solution is excreted in 6 hours and 70% in 24 hours. It is thus not so valuable as a plasma expander. But, in view of the low molecular weight passes through the capillaries more easily, decreases the blood viscosity and brings "segregated" red cells back into circulation. It is probably most effective when the circulating blood volume has been restored but shock is still present, as in transfusion resistant shock cases.

(e) Other Solutions

Some of which are being produced at present are Gelatin, Polyvinyl pyrrolidone (PUP), hydroxethyl starch etc. These are not in common use and for fuller information see Gruber (1969).

REFERENCES

Cournand, A., Riley, R. L., Bradley, S. E., Breed, E. S., Noble, R. P., Lauson, H. D., Gregerson, M. L. and Richards, D. W. (1943). Studies of the circulation in clinical shock. *Surgery*, **13**, 964.

Guyton, A. C. (1963). Circulatory Physiology: Cardiac output and its regulation. W. B. Saunders Co., Philadelphia.

Shoemaker, W. C. (1967). Shock. Charles C. Thomas, Springfield, Illinois. U.S.A.

Crowell, J. W. and Guyton, A. C. (1961). Evidence favouring a cardiac mechanism in irreversible haemorrhagic shock. *Ann. J. Physiol.* **201**, 893.

Catchpole, B. N., Hackel, D. B. and Simeone, F. A. (1955). Coronary and Peripheral blood flow in experimental haemorrhagic hypertension treated with 1-nor-epinephrine. *Ann. Surg.* **142**, 372.

Prout, W. G. (1968). Relative value of central-venous-pressure monitoring and blood-volume measurement in the management of shock. *Lancet* **1**, 611.

McGowan, G. K. and Walters, G. (1965). A clinical study of surgical shock. *Lancet* **1**, 611.

Gauer, O. H. and Henry, J. P. (1963). Circulatory basis of fluid volume control. *Physiol. Rev.* **43**, 423.

Walker, W. F., Zilcli, M. S., Reutter, F. W., Shoemaker, W. C., Friend, D. and Moore, F. D. (1959a). Adrenal medullary secretion in haemorrhagic shock. *Amer. J. Physiol.* **197**, 773.

Hume, D. M. and Nelson, D. H. (1954). Adreno-cortical function in surgical shock. *Proc. Congr. Surg. Forum Amer. Coll. Surgeons.* Philadelphia, Saunders 1955, p. 568.

Hume, D. M. and Nelson, D. H. (1954). Adreno-cortical function in surgical shock. *Proc. Congr. Surg. Forum Amer. Coll. Surgeons* Philadelphia.

Walker, W. F., Shoemaker, W. C., Kaalstad, A. J. and Moore, F. D. (1959b). Influence of blood volume restoration and tissue trauma on cortico-steroid secretion in dogs. *Amer. J. Physiol.* **197**, 781.

Dietzman, R. H. and Lillehei, R. C. (1969). Unpublished data quoted from— The nature and treatment of shock. *Brit. J. Hosp. Med.* **1**, 300, 1968.

Shoemaker, W. C. and Walker, W. F. (1969). Fluid-electrolyte therapy in acute illness. Year Book Med. Publishers.

Cohn, J. D., Greenspam, N., Goldstein, C. R., Gudwin, A. L., Siegel, J. H. and Del Guercio, L. R. M. (1968). Arterovenous shunting in high cardiac output shock syndromes. *Surg. Gynec. Obstet.* **127**, 282.

Duff, J. H., Groves, A. C., McLean, A. P. H., La Pointe, R., and MacLean L. D. (1969). Defective oxygen consumption in septic shock. *Surg. Gynec. Obstet.* **128**, 1051.

Blaisdell, F. W., Lim, R. C. and Stallone, R. J. (1970). Mechanism of pulmonary damage following traumatic shock. *Surg. Gynec. Obstet.* **130**, 15.

Shires, T., Williams, J., Brown, F. (1961). Acute changes in extracellular fluid associated with major surgical procedures. *Ann. Surg.* **154**, 803.

Shires, T. (1967). Shock and metabolism. *Surg. Gynec. Obstet.* **124**, 284.

Crocker, M. C. (1968). Blood Transfusion. A review. Anaesthesia **23**, 413.

Dudley, H. A. F., Knight, R. J., McNeur, J. C. and Rosengarten, D. S. (1968). Civilian Battle Casualties in South Vietnam. *Brit. J. Surg.* **55**, 332.

Aviado, D. M., Jnr. and Schmidt, C. F. (1955). Reflexes from stretch receptors in blood vessels, heart and lungs. *Physiol. Rev.* **35**, 247.

Smith, L. L. and Moore, F. D. (1962). Refractory hypotension in man— Is this irreversible shock? *New Eng. J. Med.* **267**, 733.

Hardaway, R. M. (1965). Intravascular coagulation in irreversible shock. Shock and Hypotension, 621, ed. L. C. Mills and J. H. Moyer, Grune & Statton, New York.

Nickerson, M. (1955). Factors of vasoconstriction and vasodilation in shock. *J. Michigan M. Soc.* **54**, 45.

Lillehei, R. C., Longereeam, J. K., Bloch, J. H. and Manax, W. G. (1964). The nature of irreversible shock. *Ann. Surg.* **160**, 682.

Murdoch, J. C. M., Speirs, C. F. and Pullen, H. (1968). The bacteraemic shock syndrome. *Brit. J. Hosp. Med.* **1**, 346.

Shoemaker, W. C. (1968). Emergency management of acute injury and shock. *Medical Times* **96**, 598.

Brooks, D. K., Williams, W. G., Manley, R. W. and Whiteman, P. (1963). Osmolar and Electrolyte changes in haemorrhagic shock. Hypertonic solutions in the prevention of tissue damage. *Lancet* **1**, 521.

Shires, T., Coln, D., Carrico, J. and Light-Foot, S. (1964). Fluid therapy in haemorrhagic shock. *Arch. Surg.* **88,** 688.

MacLean, L. D. (1968). Shock and metabolism. *Surg. Gynae. Obstet.* **126,** 299.

Eiseman, B. (1967). Combat casualty management in Vietnam. *J. Trauma,* **7,** 53.

Hardaway, R. M., James, P. M., Anderson, R. W., Bredenberg, C. E. and West, R. L. (1967). Intensive study of treatment of shock in man. *J. Amer. Med. Ass.* **199,** 779.

Walker, W. F. (1965). Blood substitutes for transfusion. *Practitioner* **195,** 187.

Gruber, U. F. (1969). Blood replacement. Springer-Verlag, Berlin.

Ross, B. A., Lord Brock and Aynsley-Green, A. (1969). Observations on central and peripheral temperatures in the understanding and management of shock. *Brit. J. Surg.* **56,** 877.

Ibsen, B. (1967). Treatment of shock with vasodilators measuring skin temperature on the big toe. Ten years' experience in 150 cases. *Dis. Chest* **52,** 425.

6: Hydrogen Ion Regulation

The term hydrogen ion regulation is used here as synonomous with the older one of acid-base balance and is concerned with the regulation of the hydrogen ion (H+) in body fluids. There is, of course, great clinical interest in this as humans are acid producers, and the end products of tissue metabolism are H+ and carbon dioxide (CO_2). Situations occur where these cannot be eliminated in the usual manner and their accumulation may produce metabolic and cardiac problems.

This was perhaps hinted at by the older medical investigators such as O'Shaughnessy (1831) who pointed out the great loss of alkali in the stools of patients with cholera, and more strongly, by Sellards (1910) who noted the large amount of alkali required to be given intravenously to cholera patients to render the urine alkaline.

These early observations bore fruit in succeeding years with the introduction of acceptable terminology and more precise and readily available methods of measurement. Even now there are still problems in the interpretation of the parameters measured and in what constitutes the primary and the secondary changes in complex metabolic disorders. Some of these problems were highlighted at a recent conference in New York (Nahas, 1966).

Basic Considerations

1. Acids and Bases

The Bronsted–Lowry system, which takes into account the central role of water in acid-base reactions, is the most acceptable. This defines an Acid as a proton donor and a Base as a proton acceptor.

Common Acids	Bases
(H+) or PROTON DONORS	(H+) or PROTON ACCEPTORS
H_2CO_3	HCO^-_3 $+H^+$
NH_4	NH_3 $+H^+$
H_2PO_4	HPO_4 $+H^+$
HCl	Cl^- $+H^+$
Lactic Acid	Lactate $+H^+$

2. Production of H^+ and CO_2

The pH of the body fluids may be lowered by the accumulation of H^+ or "potential" H^+ i.e. CO_2. This may be regarded as "potential"

H^+ because, in its transport through the body it forms an acid H_2CO_3 and if the CO_2 is not eliminated by the lungs, the ratio of H_2CO_3/HCO_3 is raised indicating increased H^+ concentration in the plasma.

(a) Source of H^+ (50–100 mEq/day)

The primary source of metabolic H^+ is the complete metabolism of proteins. These produce the mineral acids sulphuric (H_2SO_4) and phosphoric (HPO_3) as well as some organic acids. The H^+ from this source is non-volatile, and amounts to only about 50–100 mEq/day (1 mEq/Kg/day) which must be excreted in the urine.

The secondary source is the incomplete oxidation of carbohydrate and fat which should normally be oxidised to CO_2 and water. But if oxidation is incomplete as in diabetes or in states of tissue hypoxia, organic acids are produced such as pyruvic, lactic, β hydroxybutyric and aceto-acetic. As it is non-volatile, H^+ must be excreted by the kidney as ammonium ions or with buffer as titratable acidity.

(b) Source of "potential" H^+ — CO_2 (15,000 mEq/day)

CO_2 is produced by the tissues from the complete combustion of carbohydrate, fat and protein, which are finally oxydised to CO_2 and water. The production of CO_2 is massive amounting to 15,000 mEq/day. It is excreted, in its volatile form, by the lungs whose function is therefore of great importance in the regulation of the pH of the body.

3. Buffers

A solution is said to be "buffered" when it resists a change in pH even when acidic or alkaline substances are added to it. The buffering capacity of the solution is due to substances within it which can interact with acids or bases so minimising alterations in the number of free H^+ in the body fluids.

In the body these buffers are present in:—

(a) Blood: The two important buffer systems are:—

    (i) Bicarbonate/carbonic acid system, where

$$HCO^-_3 + H^+ \rightleftharpoons H_2CO_3 \rightleftharpoons H_2O + CO_2 \text{ (excreted by lungs)}$$

and (ii) Haemoglobin, main buffer action of which, is in the carriage of CO_2 from the tissues to the lung in the form of carbonic acid. $H^+ + Hb^- \rightleftharpoons HHb$.

Reduced haemoglobin is a stronger base than oxyhaemoglobin, and will therefore buffer more H^+ ions.

    (iii) Other buffers in the blood are the proteins which have about one third of the buffering power of haemoglobin and phosphates which have a smaller action still.

(b) ECF. The main buffer system here is the above mentioned, bicarbonate/carbonic acid one.

(c) ICF. The buffers in the tissue cells are proteins and inorganic phosphate.

The blood buffers, although extremely important, represent only about 20% of the buffering capacity of the body. The other 80% is in tissue cells and the E.C.F. which have roughly equal buffering capacity. Thus acids produced by cell metabolism are neutralised partially by the intracellular buffers then passing into the E.C.F. by the buffers therein and finally by the blood buffers before being excreted by the lungs or kidneys. In the reverse direction, acids added to the blood-stream are neutralised in the blood, E.C.F. and I.C.F. Excess of hydroxyl or bicarbonate ions is a much less frequent occurrence and less easily dealt with. The hydroxyl ions unite with CO_2 to form bicarbonate. The surplus bicarbonate is excreted in the urine.

4. Excretion of H^+ and CO_2

On the integrity of this depends the reaction of the body fluids. As CO_2 production is so great, ventilatory insufficiency can rapidly lead to H^+ accumulation with acidosis. The renal excretory mechanism is slower so that with renal dysfunction the accumulation of H^+ is gradual and acidosis delayed.

(a) Respiratory Control

The function of the lungs in control of the acid-base state is in its stabilisation of the partial pressure of CO_2 (PCO_2) and through it the concentration of carbonic acid (H_2CO_3) in the plasma. The CO_2 liberated from tissue cells as the end product of metabolism passes easily through the cell membrane into the interstitial fluid and from there into the plasma where it comes in contact with the red blood cells. It passes into the red cell where through the action of carbonic anhydrase it combines with water to form H_2CO_3. This dissociates into H^+ and HCO_3^-. The HCO_3^- diffuses back into the plasma in exchange for Cl^- which moves into the red cell—the "Chloride shift". In the lungs the reverse process occurs and the CO_2 liberated is passed into the alveoli. The Cl^- passes into the plasma and HCO_3 enters the red cells. It is essential for the process that the airway is clear, the alveolar epithelium is permeable to the gases, and that the alveolar ventilation is under the control of PCO_2. The latter feed back mechanism is efficient and works through the effect of PCO_2 on the respiratory centre. If the PCO_2 increases by 10 mmHg there will be a marked increase in ventilation. The respiratory centre is also sensitive to change in pH—a fall in pH of 0·1 unit can double the respiratory rate; a rise would have the opposite effect. Thus the lungs can attempt to compensate for a metabolic acidosis by producing a respiratory alkalosis.

(b) Renal Excretory Mechanism

Even when the blood pH is low there are very few free H^+ in the plasma. Robinson (1961) estimated that at a pH 7·0 the actual concentration of H^+ would only be 0·0001 mEq/1. The rest of H^+ are buffered. The problem, for the body, is to get rid of a few free H^+ and a lot of buffered H^+. This is accomplished in a number of ways resulting in a normal urine pH of 5·5–6·5. In acidosis it may be 4·5 and in alkalosis 7·8.

(i) *Filtration.* About 3 mEq of bicarbonate appear in the glomerular filtrate every minute but practically none appears in the urine. Most of it is reabsorbed to maintain the plasma HCO^-_3 but some is available to neutralise any free H^+ in the filtrate or H^+ secreted by the tubular epithelium.

(ii) *Renal Tubular Cell Activity.* This involves the hydration of CO_2 with aid of carbonic anhydrase.

$$CO_2 + H_2O \xrightarrow{\text{carbonic anhydrase}} H^+ + HCO^-_3$$

The H^+ is excreted by the tubular epithelium into the tubular lumen and HCO^-_3 passes back into the plasma. The secreted H^+ may react in three ways. First as mentioned above it may combine with HCO_3^-

$$H^+ + HCO_3^- = H_2CO_3 = H_2O + CO_2$$

A second reaction is combination with phospate
$H^+ + Na_2HPO_4 = NaH_2PO_4 + Na$ (which exchanges with the H^+ and passes into the plasma).

The H_2PO_4 is excreted as titratable acidity.

Finally H^+ may combine with ammonia (NH_3) to form ammonium (NH_4^+). The ammonia is synthesised by the distal tubular cells from glutamine and amino-acids.

(iii) *Effect of PCO_2.* The PCO_2 probably affects the renal tubular cells by changing the pH of the cell to the acid side. The cell then excretes H^+ into the tubule. A high PCO_2 increases the H^+ output in the urine: a low PCO_2 reduces H^+ output. In this way the kidney compensates for respiratory disturbances although it is a slow process.

(iv) *Paradoxical Aciduria.* Normally when the plasma pH is high indicating a state of alkalosis the urine pH should also be high. Occasionally an acid urine is excreted in the presence of alkalosis. This paradoxical state is seen in patients with pyloric stenosis, following operation, or in those on steroid therapy, and is due to one of two causes. The first is a low plasma potassium which renders the cells acid as the K^+ in the cell is replaced by H^+. The acid tubular cells thus will excrete H^+, into the tubular fluid in exchange for Na^+, producing an acid urine. If potassium is supplied to these patients intravenously the urine will again become alkaline and the alkalosis will be corrected. The second cause of the aciduria is severe sodium deficiency. A critical point occurs when sodium must be conserved otherwise hypotension will develop. The tubular Na^+ is then reabsorbed avidly in exchange for H^+.

7. Inter-relationship (*Kidney and Lungs*)

This is expressed in the well-known Henderson–Hasselbalch equation.

$$pH = pK + \log \frac{HCO_3^-}{H_2CO_3} \qquad \frac{\text{(Renal)}}{\text{Respiratory}}$$

pK is a constant (6·1) for carbonic acid.

HCO_3^- (24 mmol/L) is the base whose excretion is regulated by the kidneys. H_2CO_3 is the acid whose excretion is regulated by the lungs. For each mmHg rise in pressure of CO_2, 0·03 ml of CO_2 is dissolved in plasma.

$$
\begin{aligned}
H_2CO_3 &= pCO_2 \times \text{solubility factor for } CO_2 \\
&= 40 \times 0\cdot03 \\
&= 1\cdot2 \\
\therefore pH &= 6\cdot1 + \log \frac{24}{1\cdot2} \\
&= 6\cdot1 + \log 20 \\
&= 6\cdot1 + \log 1\cdot3 \\
&= 7\cdot4
\end{aligned}
$$

Terminology of H^+ homeostasis

The term of pH was introduced by Sorensen (1909) who developed the first electrode capable of measuring the concentration of H^+ in a solution. pH as expressed at the present time is the negative logarithm of the activity of H^+. This logarithmic expression is used to avoid the cumbersome one of 0·000040 mEq/L which corresponds to a pH of 7·40, the accepted normal figure.

The range compatible with life is 6·8–7·7. While this may not appear large it should be remembered that it is in logarithmic terms. If we change to what is perhaps a better system of quantitation that of millemicroequivalents ($m\mu Eq/L$) or nanomoles (nmol/L) the range 6·8–7·7 becomes 160–20 $m\mu Eq/L$. This is evidently a large range, much greater than that allowed for any other ion. The normal pH 7·40 becomes 40 $m\mu Eq/L$ with a normal range of 36–44 $m\mu Eq/L$ (Campbell et al, 1963).

Measurement of pH of the blood

This is usually measured in arterial blood collected anaerobically or on arterialised capillary blood collected from the ear or in case of an

infant, from a heel stab. Large amounts of blood are not required
since the development of the microtechnique using the Astrup method
and Radiometer apparatus (Fig. 29). Venous blood can be used
especially if taken from a central vein without stasis. The result is
usually 0·01–0·04 pH units below the arterial pH. A single determination on venous blood is of little value, but multiple serial

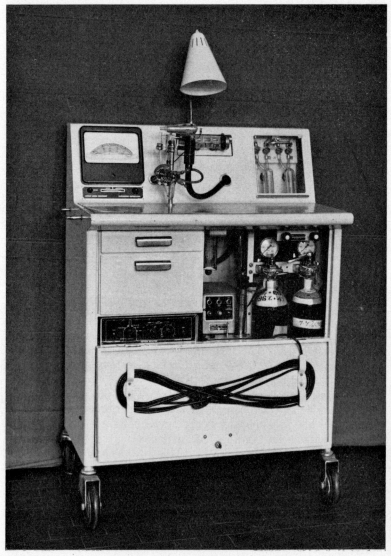

FIG. 29. Astrup machine.

estimations allow a reasonable idea of the progress of the acid/base state. In the microtechnique the finger, ear or heel is warmed and stabbed to obtain an even flow of blood in drops. A capillary tube is used to collect the blood anaerobically. The ends of the tube are

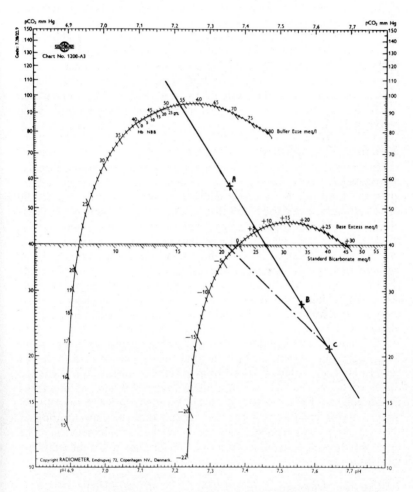

FIG. 30. Nomogram illustrating a case.

sealed with modelling wax to prevent the entry of air and the tube can be transported a distance for the measurement. The blood from an artery or vein is collected into a heparinised syringe. The needle can then be inserted into a cork or twisted to block the lumen and keep air out.

At the machine the blood is sucked up into the electrode system and the pH is measured. The blood is now equilibrated with two gases of known PCO_2 and the pH is measured again after each equilibration. With these results and using a nomogram (Fig. 30) the remaining acid/base values, namely pCO_2, base excess, or standard bicarbonate can be calculated. The blood should be fully saturated with oxygen. If it is not, corrections must be made on the nomogram. This applies also to changes in the haemoglobin concentration and temperature of the blood.

Measurement of Intracellular pH

The complexity of an ordinary cell with its heterogenous collection of organelles, mitochondria, Golgi complex, nucleus and cytoplasm gives the term cell pH a questionable meaning. Does it refer to the pH of all parts of the cell? Do they in fact have the same pH? These questions cannot at present be answered completely, but a good review of the problem was given by Bittar (1964). Certainly pH measurements of cells can be obtained by glass micro-electrodes (Caldwell, 1954), or by constructing a CO_2 dissociation curve in a tissue e.g. frog muscle (Fenn, 1928), or by using a de-methylated metabolite of Tridione (D.M.O.) (Waddel and Butler, 1959). It has been shown using these methods that the intracellular pH of most animal tissues and cells is about 7·0. In a review of the problem Waddell and Bates (1969) stated that the intracellular water was very sensitive to acidification from increasing tension of CO_2 but that highly ionised acids or bases such as HCL or $NaHCO_3$ added to extracellular water had a negligible direct effect on the pH of intracellular water. Where simultaneous measurements of pH, Na and K have been made in E.C.F. and I.C.F. under varying conditions it has been found that the concentration of these in both compartments increase or change simultaneously. The exact way in which this is accomplished is not known nor indeed is the mechanism for control of intracellular pH.

1. Carbon Dioxide Tension ($PCO_2 = 40$ mmHg)

This can be measured using a special pCO_2 electrode (Severinghaus and Bradley, 1958) or the interpolation method using the micro-Astrup apparatus may be preferred.

Changes in pCO_2 of the blood reflect the respiratory component: a low pCO_2 indicates a respiratory alkalosis due to overbreathing: a raised pCO_2 a respiratory acidosis due to underventilation as in various respiratory distress syndromes. It should be remembered that as the pCO$_2$ rises there is some dissolved CO$_2$ in the plasma. Thus the total CO$_2$ of the blood will vary with the pCO$_2$.

2. Standard Bicarbonate (HCO_3^- – 24 mEq/l)

This is defined as the plasma bicarbonate concentration after equilibration of whole blood fully oxygenated to a pCO$_2$ of 40 mmHg at 37°C and is calculated from nomograms. By standardising the respiratory component (PCO$_2$) this is taken to represent the metabolic component of an altered acid-base state. Other parameters related to this are:— The plasma CO$_2$ content (TCO$_2$) which is the toal amount of CO$_2$ present in all forms in the plasma at the actual PCO$_2$ of the blood; and the plasma bicarbonate concentration which is the concentration of bicarbonate at the actual PCO$_2$ of the blood, i.e. TCO$_2$ minus dissolved CO$_2$ in the plasma. This can be measured by the autoanalyser.

3. Whole Blood Base Excess ($BE \pm 2$)

The term Buffer Base (42–55 mEq/L) was devised by Singer and Hastings (1942) to include bicarbonate and other buffer anions especially proteinate ions. It is therefore independent of PCO$_2$ but does depend on the protein and haemoglobin concentration of the blood. By adding acid and bases to blood and calculating pH, PCO$_2$, Buffer base, etc., Anderson et al (1960), were able to construct nomograms from which the above could be calculated under varying conditions. A further calculation of Base Excess was possible which is defined as the difference between the actual Buffer Base and the normal Buffer Base. A positive value indicates a Base Excess (metabolic alkalosis), a negative value a Base deficit (metabolic acidosis). The value of this measurement of Base Excess is that it gives in quantitative terms i.e. mEq/L blood the surplus amount of fixed acid or base. From this one can calculate the amount of alkali or acid required to restore the pH to normal according to a formula (Mellemgaard and Astrup, 1960) e.g. if the Base deficits -10. This is -8 below the lower limit of normal and indicates a severe acidosis.

$$
\begin{aligned}
\text{Amount of NaHCO}_2 \text{ required} \ &= \ \text{Base deficit} \times \text{E.C.F.} \\
&= \ 10 \times (20\% \times \text{Body Weight in Kg}) \\
&= \ 10 \times 0{\cdot}2 \times 70 \\
&= \ 140 \text{ mEq.}
\end{aligned}
$$

This is most probably an underestimate as it does not take into account the H$^+$ in the cells. For this reason some multiply the total figure by 2 which approximates to the volume of the I.C.F. compartment.

Disorders of H$^+$ Homeostasis

Various classifications have been offered to characterise disorders in acid base balance. These have been thought necessary because there may be an increase in the acid load in the body which, being taken up by the buffers, is not shown by an alteration in pH. This is, by some, termed acidosis and is characterised by a normal pH and a diminished HCO_3^-. When the buffers are swamped and the pH falls this is termed acidaemia. The converse is true of alkalosis and alkalaemia. Our own view is that this is clinically an unnecessary division. We accept therefore two terms, Acidosis and Alkalosis, as being an increase in the acid or alkali load in the body or a diminution of the alkali or acid load whether the pH changes or not. Changes in these two classes are brought about by changes in carbonic acid which is under respiratory control, or in metabolic acids or alkalis.

Acidosis pH ↓

This is defined here as an increase in acid in the body or a diminution in base with alteration in acid-base ratio. It is subdivided into:—

(a) Respiratory Acidosis pH ↓ PCO_2 ↑ HCO_3^- ↑→

This is due to diminished ventilation or poor exchange of gases in the alveoli. Obviously any condition that severely impairs lung function may be implicated. A list of these is given in Table 26. This disturbance

Table 26.

Causes of Respiratory Acidosis

Airway obstruction Bronchial secretions	} Air Passages
Lack of Alveolar Surfactant Hyaline Membrane Disease Emphysema	} Alveolar Level
Pulmonary Hypertension Pulmonary Oedema Consolidation Contusion	} Interstitium
Pneumothorax Haemothorax	} Pressure on Lungs
Fractured ribs ± Flail chest Respiratory paralysis Respiratory centre failure Ventilator problems	} Chest movement problems

is reflected by a rise in PCO_2. The basic pattern is thus a fall in pH and a rise in PCO_2 along with this there is usually a rise in HCO_3^-. There are two reasons for this.

(a) An increase in dissolved CO_2 in the plasma. For each mmHg rise 0·03 ml of CO_2 is dissolved in the plasma. This is however a very small fraction of the increase in HCO_3^- observed.

(b) The buffering mechanism:— CO_2 enters the red cells where $H_2CO_3 \rightarrow H^+ + HCO_3^-$. The H^+ is buffered by haemoglobin and HCO_3 passes into the plasma in exchange for Cl—the "Chloride Shift".

The rise in PCO_2 stimulates the respiratory centre to increase the respiratory rate and depth—which helps to remove the CO_2. The action of PCO_2 in renal tubular cells has already been mentioned (p. 128)— a compensatory mechanism. The total buffer base is not affected however as the raised HCO_3^- is balanced by the decrease in haemoglobin buffer.

The electrolyte changes are: a raised HCO_3^-; a possible rise in K^+ due to extracellular shift; a normal Na^+; and a fall in Cl due to intracellular shift and renal excretion. If the respiratory acidosis remains uncorrected and is severe and no oxygen is administered, the partial pressure of oxygen will fall (PO_2) as will oxygen saturation. The tissue anoxia produced gives rise to metabolic acidosis as detailed later.

Treatment

This is centred on improving lung function. It may involve clearance of the airway passages by pharyngeal or bronchoscopic suction, tracheal intubation or tracheostomy, oxygen inhalation, and if necessary mechanical ventilation. These and the use of drugs to liquefy secretions or promote expectoration and the great value of physiotherapeutic measures are discussed in the appropriate chapter (p. 157). Carbon dioxide is more readily diffusible than oxygen so that the problem is really one of ventilatory efficiency.

(b) Metabolic Acidosis pH ↓ PCO_2 ↓ HCO_3^- ↓ K^+ ↑

This is due to the "addition" of acids or the "subtraction" of base. Various conditions in which it may occur are listed in Table 27. Initially the "addition" acids are dealt with by dilution in the body fluids, but more especially by the buffers as already detailed. Reaction of the acid

Table 27.

Causes of Metabolic Acidosis

Hypoxia	{	Cardiac
		Respiratory
Low tissue blood flow	—	Circulatory failure
Diabetes		
Renal Disease		
Drugs, e.g. NH_4Cl Salicylates, carbonic anhydrase inhibitors		
Intestinal base loss	{	Diarrhoea
		Fistulae pancreatic

with HCO_3^- liberates CO_2 which is excreted by the lungs: the plasma HCO_3^- therefore falls. Some of the acid shifts into the cells where it is buffered by intracellular buffers with shift of Ca^+, K^+ and PO_4 out of the cells. H^+ moves very slowly through the cell membrane which is freely permeable to CO_2. The renal mechanisms come into play with excretion of an acid urine. Much of the acid load is excreted with the cations Na^+, K^+, Mg^{++} and Ca^{++} and in a severe prolonged metabolic acidosis the body content of these may be diminished. Usually, however, the excretion of K^+ does not keep up with its passage from the cells into the E.C.F. and hyperkalaemia is a dangerous complication of metabolic acidosis leading to heart irregularity and death.

In subtraction acidosis i.e. loss of base as happens in severe diarrhoea, the problem is not only the accumulation of H^+ but also loss of the anion HCO_3^- which must be replaced.

Treatment of Metabolic Acidosis

This obviously depends on the cause. The extent of the dehydration should be estimated and the intake, to be given, calculated from this, the amount required for normal replacement, and for continuing losses (p. 17). Sodium bicarbonate is required to combit the acidosis; the amount required is based on frequent estimates of the acid base parameters. Hyperkalaemia will usually diminish with correction of the acidosis and the re-entry of potassium into the cells. If not, then the various measures for dealing with this should be considered (p. 35). When metabolic acidosis is due to circulatory failure as in shock, bicarbonate infusion forms a part of the overall treatment of the shock state. Blood volume replacement comes first, acid base correction second. The only area of dissention from this view is in cardiac arrest due to hyperkalaemia where HCO_3^- should be infused rapidly pari passu with cardiac massage and volume replacement.

(c) Mixed Respiratory and Metabolic Acidosis $pH \downarrow$ $PCO_2 \uparrow$ $HCO_3^- \downarrow$

Mixed acidosis is not uncommon in surgical patients, and is due to the association of respiratory and cardiovascular failure problems occurring at the same time.

It is seen therefore most commonly in shock but also in such an innocent physiological event as in the newborn who may manifest this shortly after birth for a brief period of time.

The mixed acidosis state is one to be viewed with some concern and one requiring energetic treatment of the shock and the respiratory failure. Both of these are being seen more and more often with the increase of road traffic accidents. The correction of the acidotic state becomes, in these, only one factor for correction in a programme of clinical care.

Alkalosis pH ↑ PCO_2 ↘ HCO_3^- ↑

This is defined as a decrease in the acid in the body or an accumulation of base. It is further classified as respiratory and metabolic according to the main factor responsible.

(d) *Respiratory Alkalosis pH* ↑ PCO_2 ↓ HCO_3^- ↘

This is due to overventilation with excretion by the lungs, of larger amounts of CO_2 than normal. Obviously the controlling mechanism for correcting the respiratory rate by the plasma PCO_2 has been altered. Usually it is seen in hysterical overventilation, sometimes with tetany. Occasionally it may occur in association with pain or fear in the post-operative period. Relief of pain by drugs may then abolish it. Less commonly it may be produced by unsuspected overventilation either by hand inflation by the anaesthetist or by incorrectly set mechanical ventilators. Other causes of hyperventilation are salicylate poisoning, thyrotoxicosis, severe infections, high altitudes and C.N.S. lesions.

Loss of CO_2 diminishes H_2CO_3 and as there is no loss of HCO_3^- the normal $\dfrac{HCO_3^-}{H_2CO_3}$ ratio of $\dfrac{20}{1}$ is disturbed with therefore a rise in pH or fall in H^+ concentration of the plasma. Two mechanisms operate to limit this: the first being Cations. A particularly important one is K^+ which passes into the tissue cells with Cl^- (from the R.B.C.'s) and lactate from the muscle cells passing into the E.C.F. These react with the HCO_3^- to convert it into CO_2, which is blown off reducing the HCO_3^- level in the plasma. The second mechanism is renal compensation where there is excretion of an alkaline urine containing much HCO_3^-. The depression of renal reabsorption of HCO_3^- is said to be connected closely with a falling PCO_2 (Pitt, 1963). The electrolyte changes apart from a fall in HCO_3^- are a decrease in Na^+ and K^+ and PO_4^-, either from intracellular shift or renal excretion. Ionised calcium may also fall with the onset of tetany.

The really important effect of respiratory alkalosis is on the cerebral circulation where vasoconstriction occurs in response to a low pCO_2. The fall in K^+ is not as great as in metabolic alkalosis. The tetany is easily recognised and treated.

Treatment

The initiating cause must first be determined. Psychic hyperventilation is easily cured by either breathing into a paper bag, by reassurance or by sedation. Carbon dioxide may also be administered by face mask or nasal catheter. If the K^+ level is very low then potassium supplements will be required.

(e) Metabolic Alkalosis $pH \uparrow$ $PCO_2 \downarrow$ $HCO_3^- \uparrow$ $K^+ \downarrow$

This is most commonly due to loss of H^+ and Cl^- in gastric juice from vomiting as in pyloric stenosis, high intestinal obstruction, or in gastric suction. Occasionally it results from potassium depletion the recognition of which is most important with regard to treatment. "addition alkalosis" may occur with excess bicarbonate therapy either in treatment of peptic ulcers or in overtreatment of metabolic acidosis. A further cause is massive blood transfusions causing citrate intoxication.

The main body defence mechanism against metabolic alkalosis is the renal excretion of HCO_3^-. Pitt and his colleagues (1963) found that the kidneys normally reabsorb 24–28 mEq HCO_3^- per litre of glomerular filtrate thus stabilising the plasma HCO_3^- at 24–28 mEq/L. Any HCO_3^- in excess of that is excreted in the urine. An increase in PCO_2 or decrease in intracellular K^+ both enhance HCO^-_3 reabsorption probably through the same mechanism i.e. and acid renal tubular cell. Diminished HCO_3^- absorption was noted in acute respiratory alkalosis, carbonic anhydrase inhibition and potassium infusions (Roberts et al, 1955).

The respiratory response to alkalosis is one of decreased respiratory excretion of CO_2.

The electrolyte changes are a rise in HCO_3^-; a fall in Na^+, Cl^-, and especially K^+ in the plasma.

Treatment

Where it is due to excess alkali, no treatment is necessary other than stopping the alkali. The renal capacity to excrete large amounts of HCO_3^- is great. In alkalosis due to loss of acid replacement of Cl^- and K^+ is necessary and will be considered later. Ammonium chloride may be given intravenously as an acidifying solution but should be used with great care as ammonia is toxic. It is seldom if ever necessary as saline will convey the required Cl^- and although the plasma Na^+ may not appear low there is usually a deficiency present.

Mixed Alkalotic States

Respiratory and Metabolic Alkalosis ($pH \uparrow$ $PCO_2 \downarrow$ $HCO_3^- \uparrow$)

This is theoretically possible when a patient who is vomiting or having gastric suction at the same time starts to overventilate. Such a situation is very rare and correction of each component is obvious.

Metabolic Alkalosis and Respiratory Acidosis (pH $\uparrow$ $PCO_2 \uparrow$ $HCO_3^- \uparrow$

This may be seen in the elderly patient with pyloric obstruction and ventilatory insufficiency. Obviously efforts must be made to improve the respiratory function as well as treat the alkalosis.

Diagnosis of Acid-Base Disorders

This is based on the history of the patient's illness which may indicate the probable disorder to be expected; the signs and symptoms are sometimes helpful but often not; blood analysis is the key to diagnosis aided to some extent by urinalysis.

(a) History

Condition	Acid-Base Disorder
Chest disease or injury, shock,	Respiratory Acidosis
Diabetes, renal failure, diarrhoea	Metabolic Acidosis
Vomiting from high intestinal obstruction,	Metabolic Alkalosis
Drugs, e.g. Salicylates, Alkalis.	Produce corresponding responses.

(b) Clinical Features

It is usually difficult to diagnose a particular acid-base state from the signs and symptoms. Many of the patients are suffering from pain, anxiety, dehydration and the effect of disease, drugs or treatment.

Respiratory alkalosis due to overventilation is not usually difficult to diagnose in the hysterical patient. But if due to pain or anxiety especially after surgery the respiratory effort may not be so obvious. Paraesthesia or tetany if present indicates alkalosis.

Respiratory acidosis is associated with vasodilation in the periphery and even sweating. A decreased respiratory rate is not easy to detect. In severe cases neurological symptoms such as confusion may appear.

Metabolic alkalosis has no positive identifying signs or symptoms. The patients are usually suffering from dehydration with its associated symptomatology. Increased neuromuscular irritability is said to be present sometimes but this is doubtful. One patient seen personally was admitted to a psychiatric ward because of an extreme confusional state. His plasma Cl^- level was 58 mEq/L. Appropriate treatment returned him completely to normal.

Severe Metabolic acidosis does produce a notable change in the depth of respiration (Clowes et al, 1961). When the pH falls below 7·20 the cardiac output drops and with it the blood pressure may fall or be maintained by intense vasoconstriction. As the pH falls further circulatory failure develops and if hyperkalaemia appears a change in the E.C.G. pattern may be seen (Fig. 6). The patient becomes confused, muscular twitching may appear and finally coma develops and death occurs.

(c) Blood Analysis

The parameters especially helpful are pH, PCO_2 and either standard HCO_3^- or base excess. The changes indicative of the various disorders are shown above. These must be taken in conjunction with plasma electrolytes, plasma proteins, haemoglobin concentration and oxygen saturation or PO_2 in the assessment of a patient. It is sometimes difficult to define the primary and secondary responses in complex metabolic disorders. In the past we found the old Henderson–Davenport diagram (Davenport, 1948) useful (Fig. 31). This was based on pH and plasma bicarbonate values, and allowed a reasonable interpretation of the problem for clinical use (Walker et al, 1963, Morgan et al, 1963).

The newer nomograms of Siggaard–Andersen (1965) and Campbell et al (1968) do help in the understanding of the problems but need to be interpreted carefully along with the clinical situation. In brief,

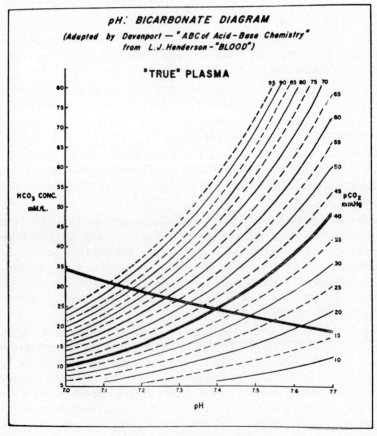

FIG. 31. ph: Bicarbonate Diagram.

there is no easy way. Critical appraisal and clear thinking with a knowledge of the basic physiology and pathology are required. A simple exposition of the acid-base balance in blood was given recently by Morgan (1969).

(d) Urinalysis

Apart from the indication this may give of underlying disease, e.g. diabetes or infection, certain measurements may be helpful. A low specific gravity in the absence of polyuria and a low urea concentration (1g/100 ml) indicates renal failure with possible renal metabolic acidosis.

In alkalosis the urine is usually alkaline pH > 7.4.

In acidosis .. .. .. acid pH < 6.0

The problem of paradoxical aciduria has already been discussed (p. 128).

Special Problems

1. Hypokalaemic Metabolic Alkalosis ($pH \uparrow \quad PCO_2 \downarrow_\rightarrow HCO_3 \uparrow \quad K \downarrow$)

The underlying cause of this condition is high intestinal obstruction, most commonly at the pylorus, with loss of the acid gastric juice. Obviously loss of highly acid juice as in peptic ulcer patients is most likely to produce the problem. Sometimes, unfortunately, the condition is produced iatrogenically by gastric suction where the acid lost is replaced by intravenous dextrose instead of normal saline. This incidentally, if continued, will give rise to water intoxication.

Vomiting of gastric contents means loss of water, H^+, Cl^-, Na^+, and K^+, in proportion to their concentration in gastric juice. Water loss results in dehydration with a fall in the E.C.F. and oliguria. Loss of H^+ and Cl^- gives rise to alkalosis. To combat this the kidneys excrete sodium and potassium bicarbonate with loss of both these cations proportional to the degree of alkalosis. The only mitigating factor is the oliguria from the dehydration. The haematocrit and blood urea rise with the onset of dehydration. The K^+ loss is accentuated by a shift from the E.C.F. into the I.C.F. In acute metabolic alkalosis this shift is probably the main mechanism for the hypokalaemia. In the more slowly developing condition both this and renal loss are operative. A third mechanism is loss by vomit but as the potassium concentration in gastric juice is only about 10 mEq/L this mechanism is not by itself very important.

Treatment

The time worn adage "to replace only that which is lost" loses none of its importance here. The intravenous therapy must be calculated according to the degree of dehydration: maintenance requirements and continuing losses. Saline with added potassium is what is required. The Na^+ and Cl^- deficit can be calculated roughly by the formula (p. 25), using E.C.F. volume for this and IBW for the K^+ deficit. As always care must be exercised in giving potassium intravenously although there is little danger if renal function is satisfactory. At the rate of 20 mEq/hour we have not observed any trouble. Repeat estimations of plasma potassium should be made and a return of this and the E.C.G. to normal allows a slowing down of the rate of infusion.

A very practical point is the timing of the operation. In pyloric stenosis there is no problem. The alkalosis and dehydration should be corrected first over a period of about 24–36 hours.

In intestinal obstruction however, a problem does exist. A frequent cause is an obstructed femoral or inguinal hernia. The fear of delay is that strangulation may be present or develop, so that operation should be carried out as soon as practically possible. Surgery will accentuate the alkalotic state as sodium will be retained and the kidneys cannot get rid of HCO_3^-. The practical course is really a compromise. Energetic measures should be taken to correct the dehydration and replace salt and potassium loss before operation, taking perhaps 6 hours to do this. The time devoted to correction will depend upon the clinical condition. For example, if the hernia is very tender, the patient toxic and strangulation likely an early operation is mandatory and a very rapid infusion over 1–2 hours should be given. The volume of saline and the potassium content should be monitored by central venous pressure (C.V.P.) and E.C.G. As in most surgical problems balanced judgment is all important.

2. Potassium depletion alkalosis ($pH \uparrow$ $PCO_2\uparrow_\rightarrow$ $HCO_3^- \uparrow$ $K \downarrow$ Urine Acid)

This is similar to the above in many ways, but differs to the extent that the emphasis is not on loss of Cl^- from the E.C.F. but on depletion of body potassium and a disturbance in the potassium gradient between the cells and E.C.F. As the E.C.F. Na^+ and Cl^- is normal or raised the treatment is replacement of potassium. Potassium depletion occurs in a variety of conditions as shown in Table 28. In the management of these salt and water are usually replaced but sometimes potassium is

Table 28.
Potassium Depletion States

1. Gastro-intestinal loss	Fistulae, diarrhoea, excessive bowel purgation.
2. Renal loss	Diuretics Adrenal Steroids Alkalosis
3. Post-operative I.V. therapy	Potassium free solutions

not. The kidney reacts to potassium depletion by reabsorbing it from the tubular fluid, but only at the expense of H^+ which, being excreted in considerable amount, render the urine acid and the plasma alkaline. The obvious corollary to this occurs in an alkalotic patient excreting an acid urine when potassium depletion should be suspected. If this is not the case then look for severe sodium deficiency.

Treatment

Potassium must be given. The amount is difficult to estimate without measuring exchangeable potassium (Ke). A rough estimate is the plasma deficit multiplied by the T.B.W. in litres. It must be controlled by serial plasma potassium estimations and the E.C.G. Saline or dextrose will be required as the vehicle depending on which is required for replacement. There is evidence that potassium alone may not, in fact, correct all cases of hypokalaemic alkalosis and that Cl^- is necessary (Aber et al, 1963, Luke and Levitin, 1967).

3. Post transfusion metabolic alkalosis

This may appear 1–3 days after massive infusions of citrated blood. These blood transfusions have two contrasting metabolic effects depending on amount of blood infused, speed of infusion and liver function. In severe shock especially where dysfunction is present the infusion of large amounts of citrated blood can even cause a metabolic acidosis. The pH falls, the plasma potassium rises and cardiac arrhythmias develop (Bunker, 1957). Where liver function is satisfactory the citrate is changed to bicarbonate and alkalosis occurs. This is usually unimportant (Litwin et al, 1959).

Recognising the effect of citrated blood on ionisable Calcium, Wolfson (1966) advised that 1 g Calcium gluconate should be given to each litre of citrated blood. Some are against routine calcium administration as they believe that the mortality from ventricular fibrillation after calcium administration is greater than in those who do not receive it (Howland, 1965).

This problem and others relative to blood replacement are excellently reviewed by Bruber, 1969.

4. Renal Acidosis ($pH \downarrow$ $PCO_2 \searrow$ $HCO_3^- \downarrow$ $K \uparrow$ $Urea \uparrow$)

This is a problem constantly in the minds of clinicians looking after patients suffering from chronic renal disease or those with severe trauma, shock, sepsis, renal calculi, or the jaundiced patient requiring surgery. Oliguria may be present after any major operation but if it persists the differential diagnosis between this and renal failure becomes important. It is further discussed on p. 173. Renal acidosis per se is due to the accumulation of H^+ due to poor ammonium excretion, and other ions such as chloride, phosphate, sulphate and organic acids.

If the plasma phosphate increases the plasma calcium may fall. Magnesium concentration may also rise but is not as important as a rise in potassium. Water accumulation dilutes the other electrolytes sodium and chloride. The rising blood urea reflects breakdown in tissue proteins and an inability to excrete nitrogen. A rapidly rising urea is seen in hyperdynamic conditions such as sepsis and severe trauma where rapid tissue breakdown is taking place.

Treatment

This is really the treatment of renal failure. Correction of the acidosis by sodium bicarbonate infusion will lessen the effects of hyperkalaemia and even help in reducing it by shifting potassium back into the cells. The treatment of hyperkalaemia is more fully discussed in chapter 2, p. 35. Briefly glucose and insulin infusion helps to lower plasma potassium. It may be removed from the body by the intestinal route using a potassium binding ion-exchange resin such as sodium polystyrene sulphonate (Resonium A) or by either peritoneal or haemodialysis. The resin can be given orally 7·5 g 4 hourly, or rectally as a daily retention enema in emulsion with cellulose and water (30 g resin, 100 ml 2% methyl cellulose, 100 ml water). (Taylor, 1965).

5. *Diabetic Acidosis pH* ↓ *PCO₂* ↗ *HCO₃⁻* ↓ *B. Sugar* ↑

Diabetes may be discovered in surgical patients especially those with severe infections or with vascular or pancreatic disease. A routine urinalysis and blood sugar estimation should prevent this being an unexpected phenomenon. But, even if suspected, surgery or infection may result in upsetting the patient's stability making it more difficult to control the condition. The acidosis is produced by accumulation of keto acids from deficient carbohydrate and fat embolism.

Treatment

This is the treatment of diabetes itself plus that of infection. Surgical intervention may actually impose the diabetic state. Sodium bicarbonate infusion will correct the pH change.

6. *Hyperchloraemic Acidosis pH* ↓ *PCO₂* ↓ *HCO₃⁻* ↓ *Cl* ↑ *K* ↓

This condition, once fairly common when uretero-sigmoidostomy was a common operation, is now becoming rather rare with the use of ileal conduits. When the ureters enter directly into the colon the back pressure due to ureteric stenosis and ascending infection can result in pyelonephritis which is in large measure the cause of the poor prognosis in these patients. The hyperchloraemia is due to urinary stasis in the colon with preferential absorption of Cl⁻ over sodium. The acidosis is increased by absorption of ammonium salts formed by urea-splitting organisms in the bowel. Normally in acidosis one expects hyperkalaemia and indeed this is sometimes present. But hypokalaemia may also occur due to loss of potassium in the urine and associated diarrhoea. It is the manifestation of either severe acidosis and/or potassium depletion which may lead to the patient's admission to hospital as an emergency.

Treatment

To some extent the condition may be prevented by daily administration of alkalinising salts such as a mixture of sodium and potassium citrate. Urinary infection must be treated. Intravenous sodium bicarbonate with added potassium is required in the emergency situation. The treatment and pathophysiology of this condition was well reviewed by Lowe et al (1959).

7. Cardiac Arrest pH $\downarrow$ PCO_2 $\uparrow$ HCO_3^- $\downarrow$

Metabolic acidosis, as has already been mentioned can lead to a fall in cardiac output and eventually cardiac arrest. It may thus ante-date the arrest or the arrest may occur from other causes and metabolic acidosis develop subsequently during the period that some circulation is going on tissue anoxia will cause metabolic acidosis. It is important therefore to stop acidosis developing by treating the incipient cardiac failure and maintaining good oxygenation and tissue blood flow. Where flow is poor sodium bicarbonate in doses of 50 mEq should be given to maintain the acid-base state until resuscitation measures are successful. Hyperkalaemia should be energetically treated. In summary emphasis should be placed on dealing with the cause of the arrest and minimising the risk of acidosis. Where arrest has occurred the first priority is to restart the heart and, if possible, correct the acidosis at the same time by infusion of bicarbonate (p. 154).

8. Open Heart Surgery pH $\downarrow$ PCO_2 $\uparrow$ HCO_3^- $\downarrow$ $\uparrow$

Cardiac patients especially the cyanotic group or those in cardiac failure may be acidotic from tissue hypoxia before operation. This should be corrected by improving the cardiac function, treating any anaemia present, and finally by an infusion of bicarbonate.

After open heart surgery respiratory acidosis commonly occurs due to hypoventilation associated with pain, overuse of drugs or retained secretions. Simple therapy will clear this up. Metabolic acidosis due to poor tissue blood flow, as a result of inadequate perfusion has disappeared largely in the simpler cases, but in the multivalvular procedures with prolonged perfusion and perhaps a temporarily depressed cardiovascular activity in the immediate post-operative period, metabolic acidosis may be seen. This is treated by improving heart action by the use of drugs such as isoprenaline and the infusion of $NaHCO_3$. Respiratory problems are also common in these patients and tracheostomy with intermittent positive pressure ventilation may be required. It is sometimes difficult to get the lungs functioning well enough to dispense with the ventilator.

9. Shock ($pH \downarrow$ $PCO_2 \uparrow\downarrow$ $HCO_3^- \downarrow$)

The acid-base changes in shock are variable. Circulatory failure will produce metabolic acidosis. Where respiratory difficulty is present respiratory acidosis will appear but in a group of shock cases we found that 6 out of 15 had overventilation with slight to moderate degree of respiratory alkalosis.

Treatment

The emphasis must be on treating the cause of the shock. Blood volume is replaced first, then acid-base disorders are corrected. Finally fluid and electrolyte disorders are sorted out.

10. Metabolic Acidosis in Burns ($pH \downarrow PCO_2 \nearrow HCO_3^-$) $\downarrow$

This problem was reviewed recently by Peaston (1968). He found in a study of 14 patients admitted to a regional burns unit that metabolic acidosis was commonly present (12 out of 14 patients). In 10 patients this was maximum on admission or within 24 hours. The degree of acidosis correlated closely with the area burned. In the severe burns a compensatory respiratory alkalosis was usually present.

Treatment

As in shock, which is usually present in burns cases of moderate to severe degree, the emphasis is on correcting blood volume deficits either present or impending due to plasma leakage; fluid replacement; correction of the metabolic acidosis and prevention of infection. Artz (1960) and Peaston (1967, 1968) feel that early correction of the metabolic acidosis with $NaHCO_3$ will do much to minimise the problems.

REFERENCES

O'Shaughnessy, W. B. (1831). Experiments on the blood in cholera. *Lancet* **1**, 490.

Sellards, A. W. (1910). Tolerance for alkalis in Asiatic cholera. *Phillipine J. Sc.*, B.5 363.

Nahas, G. G. (1966). Current concepts of acid-base balance. (Ed. Nahas, G. G.). *Ann. N.Y. Acad. Sc.* **133**, 1.

Robinson, J. R. (1961). Fundamentals of Acid-Base regulation. Blackwell Scientific Publications, Oxford.

Campbell, E. J. M., Dickinson, C. J. and Slater, J. D. H. (1968). Clinical Physiology, 3rd Ed., Blackwell Scientific Pub., Oxford.

Bittar, E. E. (1964). Cell pH. Butterworths, London.

Caldwell, P. C. (1954). An investigation of the intracellular pH of crab muscle fibres by means of micro-glass and micro-tungsten electrodes. *J. Physiol.* **126**, 169.

Fenn, W. O. (1928). The carbon dioxide dissociation curve of nerve and muscle. *Amer. J. Physiol.* **85**, 207.

Waddell, W. J. and Butler, T. C. (1959). Calculation of intracellular pH from the distribution of 5, 5-dimethyl-2, 4-oxazolidinedione (DMO). Application to skeletal muscle of the dog. *J. Clin. Invest.* **38**, 720.

Waddell, W. J. and Bates, R. G. (1969). Intracellular pH. *Physiological Review* **49**, 285.

Severinghaus, J. W. and Bradley, A. F. (1958). Electrodes for blood pO_2 and pCO_2 determination. *J. Appl. Physiol.* **13**, 515.

Singer, R. B. and Hastins, A. B. (1948). An improved clinical method for the estimation of disturbances of the acid-base balance of human blood. *Medicine Baltimore* **27**, 29.

Siggaard-Andersen, O. (1965). The acid-base status of the blood. 3rd ed. Munksgaard, Copenhagen.

Mellemgaard, K. and Astrup, P. (1960). The quantitative determination of surplus amounts of acid or base in the human body. *Scand. J. Clin. Lab. Invest.* **12**, 187.

Pitts, R. F. (1963). Physiology of the Kidney and Body Fluids. Year Book, Chicago.

Roberts, K. E., Randall, H. T., Sanders, H. L. and Hood, M. (1955). Effects of potassium on renal tubular reabsorption of bicarbonate. *J. Clin. Invest.* **34666**, 1955.

Clowes, G. H. A., Sabga, G. A., Kontitaxis, A., Tomin, R., Hughes, M. and Simeone, F. A. (1961). Effects of acidosis on cardiovascular function in surgical patients. *Ann. Surg.* **154**, 524.

Davenport, H. W. (1958). The A.B.C. of Acid-base chemistry. 4th ed. Univ. of Chicago Press, Chicago.

Walker, W. F. (1963). Biochemical changes in open heart surgery with extra corporeal circulation. *Scot. med. J.* **8**, 141.

Morgan, H. G., Ogilvie, R. R. and Walker, W. F. (1963). Acid-base monitoring in open-heart surgery. *J. Clin. Path.* **16**, 545.

Siggaard-Andersen, O. (1965). The acid-base status of the blood. 3rd ed. Copenhagen, Munksgaard.

Morgan, H. G. (1969). Acid-base balance in blood. *Brit. J. Anaes.* **41**, 196.

Aber, G. M., Sampson, P. A., Whitehead, T. P. and Brooke, B. N. (1962). The role of chloride in the correction of alkalosis associated with potassium depletion. *Lancet* **2**, 1028.

Luke, R. G. and Levitin, H. (1967). Impaired renal conservation of chloride and the acid-base changes associated with potassium depletion in the rat. *Clin. Sc.* **32**, 511.

Bunker, J. P. (1957). Citric acid intoxication. *Anaesth. Analg.* **36**, 82.

Litwin, M. S., Smith, L. L. and Moore, F. D. (1959). Metabolic alkalosis following massive transfusion. *Surgery* **45**, 805.

Wolfson, L. F. (1966). The anaesthetists management of the injured patient. *Brit. J. Anaesth.* **38**, 274.

Howland, W. S. and Boyan, C. P. (1964). Massive blood replacement without calcium administration. *Surg. Gynae. Obstet.* **118**, 814.

Gruber, U. F. (1969). Blood replacement. Spinger-Verlag, Berlin.

Taylor, W. H. (1965). Fluid therapy and disorders of electrolyte balance. Blackwell, Oxford.

Lowe, K. G., Stowers, J. M. and Walker, W. F. (1959). Electrolyte disturbances in patients with uretero-sigmoidostomy. *Scot. Med. J.* **4,** 473.

Peaston, M. J. T. (1968). Metabolic acidosis in burns. *Brit. Med. J.* **1,** 809.

Artz, C. P. (1960). Complications in Surgery and their Management. Ed. C. P. Artz & J. D. Hardy. Philadelphia.

Peaston, M. J. T. (1967). Maintenance of metabolism during intensive patient care. *Post grad. med. J.* **43,** 317.

7: Special Problems in Surgical Care

The emphasis in the earlier chapters has been on the physiological basis of surgical care. We propose now to deal with some special problems mainly from a clinical point of view. It is difficult to allocate priorities to any body system. Each is a link and the disorders of one system will often affect others. We will now consider briefly the importance, to the surgeon, of assessing normal and abnormal function. In each system emphasis will be placed on problems which may arise before or after operation.

Cardiovascular System

The basic physiology of the system has largely been dealt with in the chapter on circulatory homeostasis. Therein also the major problem of shock was discussed. Some of the common emergency conditions resulting in cardiac embarrassment in surgical patients will now be considered.

Preoperative Assessment

The detailed assessment of the cardiac patient is beyond the scope of this book. It will be sufficient to mention a few particular features that should alert the surgeon to the possibility of a disturbance in the cardiovascular system.

The importance of a history of a previous cardiac complaint, angina of effort, dyspnoea on exertion etc. is self-evident of a possible cardiac problem. Important also is the history of "little strokes" and intermittent claudication indicating peripheral vascular disease involving the cerebral or limb vessels due most likely to atheroma. If this is present in the peripheral vessels the coronary arteries may also be affected. The patient's history may indicate a hereditary predisposition to vascular disease and the presence of diabetes or excessive smoking (20/day) should cause concern.

In the routine examination of the cardiovascular system all pulses should be palpated. A full blood examination, X-ray of chest and E.C.G. should also be carried out.

Cardiac Failure

Impairment of cardiac functions leads to certain changes in the body—haemodynamic and metabolic. These may be the immediate result of failure of the pump mechanism or may, to an extent, be compensatory.

The haemodynamic changes are a fall in cardiac output usually with a drop in blood pressure and under-perfusion of the tissues. This results in metabolic acidosis which further depresses heart action and a vicious circle develops. The pulmonary venous pressure may rise and pulmonary oedema ensue. Right heart failure produces an increased venous pressure with distended neck veins, enlarged liver, and oedema of the legs leading eventually to anasarca.

The metabolic changes are consequent upon increased venous pressure causing retention of water in the tissues. This is accentuated by the diminished vis-a-tergo and increase in aldosterone secretion seen in these patients. Water is retained along with, and in excess of, salt which leads to water logging with a hypotonic state. The serum sodium and albumin falls.

Anorexia is common with therefore a deficient calorie intake. This and limited activity leads to wasting of muscle. The serum potassium may rise especially if any degree of renal failure is present. The total blood volume is increased in these patients with a fall in body cell mass and a rise in body water, especially extracellular water.

When cardiac failure is acute, the haemodynamic changes are predominant as time is required for metabolic changes to become noticeable.

Obviously operation in the presence of cardiac failure would be dangerous as the circulatory system is already stressed and the retention of salt and water would be accentuated by the response to surgery.

Treatment

If at all possible, time should be spent prior to surgery improving the condition of the patient. Salt intake should be restricted. Water and salt excretion should be encouraged by diuretics, and cardiac function improved by digitalis. It should be remembered, in this context, that diuretics increase potassium excretion so that the serum potassium may be low. Usually potassium supplements are given to prevent this and sometimes spironolactone may be used to block potassium excretion. Anaemia will require treatment by infusion of packed cells. The acid base state should be assessed and sodium bicarbonate given, if required, to correct an acidosis.

In acute cardiac failure digitalis, diuretics, oxygen therapy and morphia may all be given. In pulmonary oedema not responsive to these the over expanded blood volume may require reduction by venesection. If the heart is slow with a low blood pressure and high venous pressure Isoprenaline is useful, but its effect should be monitored on the oscilloscope as ventricular overactivity and fibrillation may be produced. If this is ineffective, cardiac pacing, external or internal, should be considered. Means of assisting the failing heart for a few hours by using extracorpeal circulation are being tried in some centres. It is too early yet to comment on their value, but there is little doubt that further work in this important field should be continued.

Cardiac Arrest

This is the most critical of all emergencies since there are only about 4 minutes, at normal temperature, in which to restart the heart. Beyond this the risk of brain damage is so great as to make its correction doubtful. To restart a heart and be left with a severely damaged brain is the greatest fear of the medical attendant.

Types of Arrest

There are 3 main types of cardiac arrest. The most common is *Ventricular Fibrillation* where there is an irregular wave-like activity over the heart muscle with no regular contractions. Besides being the commonest type, it is the most favourable—if such a term can be used in this condition—as it can be shocked back into normal rhythm by an electrical current—D.C. defibrillation. The second type is *Ventricular Standstill* or asystole when there are no contractions whatsoever and the E.C.G. is flat. Finally there is a third type of *ineffective ventricular contractions*. In this the ventricle beats regularly but with no power, so that there is virtually no output.

Patients at Risk

There are many causes of cardiac arrest and so many factors involved that a list of them is rather lengthy and indigestible.

Milstein (1967) suggested that most cases of acute circulatory arrest associated with operations, anaesthesia, and trauma were preventable. It is perhaps better, therefore, to consider the patients in whom cardiac arrest may occur if steps are not taken to prevent it.

These "at risk" patients fall mainly into the following 4 groups:—

I *Post Myocardial Infarction*

The first week after a myocardial infarct is the danger period when sudden bursts of electrical activity in the heart may trigger off ventricular fibrillation. These patients should therefore be under the closest possible supervision, if possible in a coronary care unit. It is obvious that, as all patients with heart attacks do not need this facility, selection of the worst cases could be made, and their surveilance intensified. Thus, any irregularity of rhythm can be dealt with as it arises.

II *Operation Group*

Cardiac arrest during anaesthesia is due to many causes, one of the commonest being low blood volume (Dimmick, 1964).

The emergency operation cannot always be carried out under the best conditions. But time spent in adequate preparation of the patient, restoring blood volume correcting fluids and electrolytes balance and acid/base metabolism is invaluable.

A critical time is the induction phase of anaesthesia when the unstable cardio-vascular system may react abnormally to drugs and when the risk of inhalation of stomach contents is greatest. The seriously ill surgical emergency requires the care and close co-operation of the most experienced anaesthetist and surgeon. The patient with a ruptured aortic aneurysm is especially vulnerable, as blood loss and aortic clamping all react on an already severely stressed myocardium.

III *Post-operative Group*

This naturally follows on from the previous group as factors are common to both especially the risk of inhalation of vomitus. Sudden collapse after operation is often thought to be the result of a coronary infarction occurring during the operation or immediately afterwards. This is rarely the case. An incidence of 2·3% has been reported in patients with ischaemic heart disease and hypertension (Chamberlain and Edmonds–Seal, 1964). This small percentage does not, however, indicate the possible incidence of non-fatal myocardial infarction. The routine use of the E.C.G. before, during, and after operation should be encouraged in the severely ill adult patients. Cardiac arrest following pulmonary embolism is discussed on p. 165.

IV *Miscellaneous*

There are many other causes of cardiac arrest. Especially important is the reaction to drugs. A list of those which may cause trouble has been given by McIver (1965). Electrocution is a well known cause and always a possibility in an operating theatre. Drowning and other causes are of less importance to the surgeon.

Diagnosis of Cardiac Arrest

In the majority of cases "sudden" stoppage of the heart is clinically apparent. But, this may not be a sudden event; rather the end of a gradual process of deterioration with a falling blood pressure, which may have passed unnoticed, a bradycardia and cessation of respiration.

The absence of pulses, skin circulation, respiration and blood pressure are good presumptive evidence that arrest has occurred, or, at least, that the "pump" is not working efficiently. Auscultation and finally E.C.G. leave no doubt.

Treatment

There are infinite variations in the management of such a patient. The principles however can be enumerated and there are three main ones:—

(1) Get oxygen to the alveoli
(2) Restart the "pump" action of the heart
(3) Restore the heart action to normal

These three aims of management require three phases of activity the first two of which are carried out together and are inter-dependent.

Phase I   Respiratory Phase of Activity

Under optimum conditions the airway must be cleared, if necessary by suction, the head is tilted back and an endotracheal tube is passed. In less than ideal conditions air can be administered by "mouth to mouth" breathing or better by the use of air bellows. The chest must be seen to rise and fall with respiration.

Phase II   "pump" action phase

As air or oxygen is being administered the oxygenated blood must be passed on to the tissues by restoration of the circulation. This is encouraged by cardiac massage. The patient should be lying on the floor or a firm board. External massage is preferable in nearly all circumstances using the techniques popularised by Kowenhoven et al (1960). Although the circulation is restarted by this means it is by no means as good as usual. It does however maintain life until the heart itself can be made to take over. Various mechanical aids to external massage have been produced. They certainly relieve the person compressing the chest and have been fairly successful. Internal massage produces more efficient circulation but should probably be restricted to the operating theatre. It is certainly necessary under the conditions of cardiac tamponade, intracardiac obstruction, air embolism, massive haemorrhage, or chest injury and when there is gross displacement of the heart (Milstein, 1967).

Phase III   Restoration of Cardiac Action

It is hoped that with oxygenation and mechanical stimulation of the heart from pressure, heart action will restart. If not it certainly gives time to get an E.C.G. to determine the exact type of arrest. If there is delay in getting this one may act on the assumption that ventricular fibrillation is the commonest cause of arrest and give a shock by direct current defibrillation.

If complete standstill is present the position is less hopeful. Pace-makers can be inserted intravenously but have not been very successful. Drug therapy may be helpful if the heart action does not start up spontaneously.

Drug therapy

Six drugs are used in treatment of these patients:—

1. Sodium Bicarbonate

Metabolic acidosis should be presumed in all these patients. This is known to have a bad effect on cardiac action and therefore should be corrected. Too much must not however be expected from the administration of sodium bicarbonate. It is sometimes given as 8·4% $NaHCO_3$ which amounts to 1 mEq/ml. Such a solution is not however stable and 4·2% $NaHCO_3$ is more often used. About 50 mEq $NaHCO_3$ is given to a patient and the blood removed for assessment of the acid/base state. Further titration depends on the measurements obtained.

2. Adrenaline Chloride

This has a powerful effect in increasing the power of heart action. It is usually given into the ventricles as 5–10 ml of a 1/10,000 solution.

3. Isoprenaline

It is marketed in this country as ISUPREL and has a powerful cardiotonic effect. It does, however, have a risk of causing ventricular fibrillation which may need to be corrected by the defibrillator.

4. Calcium Chloride

This is given because of its cardiotonic effect as 5–10 m of 1% Calcium Chloride. It should be used with care, if at all, in patients on digitalis or with a low serum potassium.

5. Lignocaine Hydrochloride

This anaesthetic solution has the effect of depressing irritability of the heart and is used in 25–50 mgm doses when ventricular extra systyoles are present.

6. Atropine Sulphate

Used in treatment of bradycardia due to increased vagal activity in the dose of 1·25 mgm intravenously.

When to start and when to stop

This problem in management can be an ethical one. The time between arrest and death of brain cells is short, about 4 minutes, so that damage may already be present especially in the elderly patient.

The heart may respond to the extent of an E.C.G. tracing of complexes but the cardiac output may remain very poor. Repeated defibrillation may be necessary usually with decreasing effect. How long resuscitation should continue is impossible to state precisely. The overall condition of the patient and the state of the heart itself must be considered. Dilatation of the pupils, once regarded as an absolute sign of irreversibility is now known to be valueless in patients comatose with drugs. All that can be said is that mature judgment must be exercised and each case be considered on its own merits. The decision to stop treatment should be an unanimous one on the part of the medical attendants.

Arrhythmias
Perhaps the most common irregularity is:—

Atrial Fibrillation
This is not uncommon in patients after a thoracotomy and usually corrects itself spontaneously in 2–3 days. The rate is not very rapid and circulatory embarassment is uncommon. If signs of failure develop digitalis should be given.

Atrial fibrillation is also seen in conditions, treated jointly with the physicians, such as mitral valve disease and thyrotoxicosis. In cardiac units it may be seen after mitral valvotomy and be corrected by direct shock at a specific point on the cardiac complex—cardio-version.

Ventricular Extrasystoles
These are occasionally seen on the oscilloscope in patients during operation such as resection of aortic aneurysm or in severely ill patients in the post-operative phase. They are a warning of the possibility of ventricular fibrillation and should therefore be taken seriously especially if they increase in frequency. The drug of choice is Lignocaine (1 ml/Kg) at the rate of 1 ml/min. This is given intravenously using a constant infusion pump and, as it is a depressant drug, care must be exercised in its use. Other drugs available are procaine amide, quinidine, and propanolol.

Ventricular Tachycardia
This is a run or burst of extrasystoles. If allowed to go on there is inefficient filling of the ventricles with left ventricular failure. Intravenous lignocaine may be used to control these or countershock by direct current may be necessary.

Ventricular Fibrillation
As already mentioned this is the commonest cause of cardiac arrest and its treatment has been discussed. Sometimes a sharp blow on the

precordium may restore sinus rhythm if not the D.C. defibrillator is required urgently.

Supra-Ventricular Tachycardias

Apart from atrial fibrillation these are not common in surgical cases and will therefore only be mentioned. The diagnosis is made on E.C.G. evidence and includes the following:—

Irregularity	*Treatment*
Paroxysmal atrial tachycardia	— Cardioversion
Atrial fibrillation	— Nil; Digitalis: Cardioversion
Nodal tachycardia	— Nil; Rarely cardioversion
Atrial flutter	— Digitalis

Sinus bradycardia

The slow heart rate in the surgical patient may lead to hypotension, shock, and cardiac arrest. Intravenous atropine (0·6–1·25 mgm) is usually helpful in speeding up the heart rate. If not, intracardiac pacing may be instituted.

Heart Block

The various types of heart block are usually associated with myocardial infarction. In pulmonary embolism right branch bundle block may occur and in cardiac surgery various types are seen.

Isoprenaline may be tried as a first step or while preparing for heart pacing. A dose of 2 mgm in 500 ml of dextrose is given by a constant infusion pump under E.C.G. control to raise the ventricular rate to 60 beats per minute. Further therapy should be carried out in consultation with a cardiologist.

REFERENCES

Dinnick, O. P. (1964). Deaths associated with anaesthesia; observations on 600 cases. *Anaesthesia* **19**, 536.

Chamberlain, D. A. and Edmonds-Seal, J. (1964). Effects of surgery under general anaesthesia on the electro cardiogram in ischaemic heart disease and hypertension. *Brit. Med. J.* **2**, 784.

McIver, A. K. (1965). Drug incompatability. *Pharm. J.* **195**, 609.

Milstein, B. B. (1967). Acute circulatory arrest. *Brit. J. Surg.* **54**, 471.

8: Respiratory System

Physiological Considerations

Before considering the pathological aspects of lung disorders some basic physiological principles need stating. These are, of necessity, few and are considered briefly. The classic text-books on the subject such as by Comroe et al (1962) and Nunn (1970) should be consulted for greater detail.

Ventilation—Perfusion

The interchange of respiratory gases depends on alveolar ventilation, perfusion and permeability of the alveolar membrane. Surface acting material (Surfactant) is said to act by preventing collapse of the alveoli (atelectasis) and possibly by encouraging the permeability. On the other side of the alveolar membrane is another which belongs to the capillary. Between these two membranes is a potential space which in disease states such as pulmonary oedema may actually expand to produce a barrier to the free passage of gases. Flow through the capillaries as well as alveolar ventilation are the main factors which govern the rate of interchange of the gases which, itself, is a physical process depending on differences in gas tensions across the membranes. The relationship of alveolar ventilation to pulmonary blood flow is termed the ventilation/perfusion ratio and is really the key to the understanding of pulmonary function. In the erect position the alveoli at the apex of the lung are less well ventilated than those at the base and also receive less blood flow. There is thus a linear fall in the ratio from apex to base (West 1965). As the alveolar ventilation is about 4 L/min. and the pulmonary blood flow is about 5 L/min the normal ratio is 4/5 or 0·8. In the supine position the differences in ventilation—perfusion in different parts of the lungs practically disappears.

In lung disease, with damage to the alveoli, there may be under-ventilation of some alveoli with, therefore, a reduction in arterial PO_2 and an increase in PCO_2 in the blood leaving these alveoli. The tendency for the peripheral arterial PCO_2 to rise is compensated for by over-ventilation of the non-affected alveoli and, as the dissociation curve of CO_3 is linear, so the excretion of CO_3 is directly related to alveolar ventilation. Over-ventilation will not, however, compensate for the reduction in PO_2 as blood cannot be saturated more than 100%; ventilation perfusion imbalance of this type where perfusion is normal, will produce hypoxia (PO_2) without a rise in PCO_2. Enrichment of inspired oxygen to 30% or so, will restore the arterial PO_2 to normal if no gross arterio-venous shunting is present. When ventilation and perfusion are abnormal with increase in non-functioning or under-perfused alveoli, hypoxia occurs with a rise in the PCO_2—a more serious type of respiratory failure not uncommon in surgical patients ($PO_2\downarrow$, $PCO_2\uparrow$).

Perfusion of the lungs is related to cardiac output and control of lung vessels. These react in the opposite way to systemic arterioles in that pulmonary arteriolar constriction may occur when the systemic arterioles are dilated. They can also differentially constrict in different parts of the lung producing a selective diversion of flow of blood from regions of high vascular resistance and low ventilation to others which are better ventilated and have lower resistance (McIntyre, 1969).

Respiratory Function Measurements

These are often carried out in the assessment of the patient's fitness for operation, or to study the results of lung pathology. But first we should look at the problem of lung "spaces".

Anatomical Dead Space. This is the area of the respiratory passages where gaseous exchange does not occur. It amounts, in volume of air contained, to 140 ml.

Normal Inspiration. During quiet breathing we breathe in and out about 500 ml of air. This is the TIDAL VOLUME. Of this (500 less 140 ml) 360 ml of air actually comes into contact with alveolar membrane. Thus breathing at the rate of 12 breaths/min the TOTAL ALVEOLAR VENTILATION will be 12 × 360 ml/min or 4·22 L/min.

Physiological Dead Space. This concept concerns deficiencies in circulation of blood through the lungs which cause areas to be under-perfused, with therefore an increase in the area where air is not in contact with capillaries. While this is unimportant normally, in pathological conditions the physiological dead space air may be so increased as to lead to hypoxia. This will also occur where there is adequate perfusion but no ventilation of the alveoli, as in pulmonary collapse.

Measurements

1. Volumes

The *Vital Capacity* is the volume of air expelled at maximum voluntary expiration after maximum voluntary inspiration. It is simply measured by expiring into a measuring instrument or spirometer and amounts to about 4 litres. Because of the wide range and effect of age, sex and body size which must be taken into account, it is of limited clinical value. A more commonly used measurement is the FORCED EXPIRATORY VOLUME (F.E.V.) which is the maximum volume of air the subject can expel into a spirometer. It is usually measured over 1 second (F.E.V.$_1$) when normally over 75% of the *Vital Capacity* should be expelled. The FEV$_1$ is thought to be a sensitive index of the severity of obstructive respiratory disease.

These tests may be measured before and after therapy, such as bronchodilators, to note the capacity of the obstructive lesion to improve.

2. *Flow*

A simple measurement of airway obstruction is obtained by means of the Wright peak flow meter (Wright and McKerrow, 1959). The patient blows into an instrument which has a pivoted vane controlled by a coiled spring which itself is connected to a calibrated dial. The movement of the vane is proportional to the flow rate. The maximum movement obtained on the dial on expiration is the peak flow rate (P.F.R.). The normal peak flow rate is 500 L/min.

3. *Specialised Measurements*

More complicated measurements such as lung compliance or gas transfer factor require reference to specialised respiratory units.

4. *Blood Gases*

These are the main parameters measured in the clinical assessment of respiratory function.

Oxygen. This makes up about 21% of inspired air. As it exchanges in the pulmonary capillaries with CO_2 the alveolar oxygen falls to 13·8%. But, when this is expired, the oxygen content increases to 16·4% because of the mixture with "dead space" air. Analysis of oxygen in the air is carried out rarely except experimentally, but the concentration and pressure in the blood is often measured.

The oxygen saturation of blood is measured either by a haemoreflector or less accurately by an ear oximeter. The normal oxygen saturation of actual blood is 95–98% at a normal oxygen pressure (PO$_2$) of 100 mmHg. In venous blood the saturation drops to about 74% with a PO$_2$ of 40 mmHg. A mixed venous oxygen saturation below 60% is very unsatisfactory. It should be remembered that even with very high oxygen pressures, as in the case of hyperbaric oxygen, it is impossible to saturate blood beyond 100%.

The oxygen content of the blood relates to the ability of haemoglobin to combine with oxygen. As one gram of haemoglobin can combine with 1·34 ml of oxygen, the normal content of arterial blood should be 20 ml of oxygen per 100 ml of blood. But as the blood is rarely

100% saturated the more accurate oxygen capacity for arterial blood is 19 ml per 100 ml. In venous blood the content is much smaller being about 14 ml of oxygen per 100 ml of blood.

The arterial oxygen tension is 100 mmHg. As the blood passes through the capillaries in the tissues the tension falls to about 40 mmHg —that of venous blood. During this fall in pressure the blood gives up oxygen and the oxygen capacity falls to 70%. The relationship of oxygen tension to oxygen saturation is shown in the oxygen dissociation curve (Fig. 32). Various factors effect this curve such as haemoglobin concentration, temperature, acid/base state of blood and varying oxygen pressures.

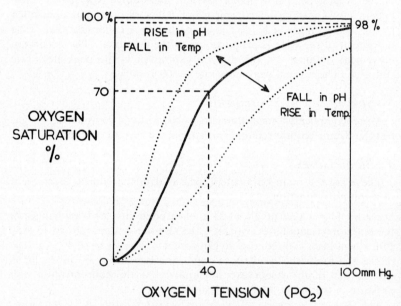

FIG. 32. Oxygen dissociation curve.

The PO_2 of blood can now be measured by a special oxygen electrode, and this can be adapted to the ASTRUP machine. It is not, however, an easy estimation, requiring continual practice to make results meaningful. As already stated the normal arterial PO_2 is 98 mmHg but it varies with age as well as disease states. In the elderly 98 mmHg would be regarded as a high normal figure. These figures become important in regard to oxygen therapy. All too often clinicians strive to maintain the pressure at the high normal level. A lower figure of 75 mmHg or even lower may be acceptable in certain cases.

Carbon Dioxide Pressure (PCO_2), as mentioned previously this can be measured directly by an electrode or deduced from a nomogram where other factors in the Henderson–Hasselbalch equation have been measured.

The normal arterial PCO_2 is 40 mmHg: the venous PCO_2 is slightly higher—46 mmHg. A rising PCO_2 indicates poor respiratory function.

Assessment of Patient for Operation

The problem often presents as an elderly patient with a long history of recurrent attacks of bronchitis who requires an operation. What complications do we look out for?

Clinical Assessment

History. There are two important points here. Firstly the progressive nature of the condition and secondly the effect of exercise. There are no precise rules to lay down. Obviously someone who has been progressively dyspnoeic and who is breathless lying flat is no fit subject for operation. If operation is mandatory attempts should be made to secure improvement in the condition by antibiotics, bronchodilators, physiotherapy and treatment of associated heart disease.

EXAMINATION. Certain features to be looked for in the examination of the chest are:—

(a) Respiratory rate and depth.

(b) Barrel-shaped chest of emphysema—use a tape measure to get expansion.

(c) Use of accessory muscles of respiration.

(d) Signs of enlarged heart.

(e) Quality of breath sounds and presence of adventitious sounds.

(f) Presence of cyanosis or finger clubbing.

Investigations

1. Plain X-ray, P.A. and lateral, are extremely helpful in eliminating gross disease.

2. Measurement of respiratory function e.g. using Wright Peak flow meter.

3. Blood gas analysis.

4. Blood analysis for anaemia.

5. Sputum analysis for tubercle bacilli and malignant cells.

6. E.C.G. for right ventricular strain.

Effect of Operation

Following any operation there is depression of lung function as a result of diminished ventilation. Factors such as apprehension, pain, tight bandages, sore throat from intubation, upper abdominal wounds, and weakness of respiratory muscles are all important. Depression of the cough reflex from the same factors plus sedation makes matters worse by causing retention of secretions. But added to these are certain fairly well defined entities which may require to be treated energetically, such as, heart disease, abdominal distension, dehydration, and heavy sedation etc. These have been reviewed in detail by Anscombe (1959). Smoking also aggravates problems in the post operative period.

Post Operative Pulmonary Complications

Acute Bronchitis. This may occur de novo or may be a flare up of a chronic bronchitic condition. There are surprisingly few signs, apart from a productive cough, a mild pyrexia of 99–100°F and possibly a few râles in lungs on ausculation.

Treatment. Breathing exercises and encouragement to cough will probably bring about a slow improvement in the condition. If there is a pyrexia, and if the sputum becomes purulent, antibiotics may be given. The choice may vary with the bacterial resistance pattern in different areas of the country, and on the sensitivity reports of sputum cultures.

Pneumonitis. The infection may spread from the bronchi to involve the lung parenchyma in the elderly or very ill patients. This is especially liable to occur in areas of collapse. The patient is now obviously ill with increased respiratory rate, fever, and tachycardia. Dullness to percussion and diminished breath sounds may be heard, with in other areas râles and rhonchi.

Treatment. Antibiotics and if necessary oxygen are the mainstay of treatment. If the pneumonitis is extensive and the situation desperate hydrocortisone may be given in large doses (500 mg every 6 hours) (Clowes, 1967).

Lung Abscess. This is a rare post-operative complication and if it does occur must reflect poorly on previous treatment. It is more often seen pre-operatively as a result of inhalation of foreign bodies, e.g. peanuts or in association with lung cancer or tuberculosis.

In the post-operative period the patient is usually very ill with a high temperature and signs and symptoms of extensive local pneumonitis. An X-ray will confirm the presence of a localised area of infection in the lung and if it connects with the air passage a fluid level may be seen.

Treatment. Consists of antibiotics and postural drainage. If it becomes chronic, excision of the abscess might be contemplated.

ATELECTASIS. This occurs usually within the first 48 hours after operation. Early clinical signs are a slight tinge of cyanosis in the lips, and either a slight increase in respiratory rate or a grunt at the end of inspiration. There may be a slight rise in temperature and increase in pulse rate. Auscultation may reveal a diminished air entry or a few crepitations in the lung bases. X-rays may show a small area of collapse. In more massive collapse the respiratory symptoms and signs are more prominent until severe respiratory failure is evident with a massive lung collapse and tracheal shift to the affected side. Shift of the mediastinum may produce cardiac embarrassment. The cause is blockage of a bronchus by a plug of mucus or by the impaction of aspirated material.

Treatment. In the milder cases percussion and postural drainage with encouragement to cough may be sufficient. In severe cases the plug must be removed by bronchoscopy and aspiration. Even in the very ill patient this life-saving manoeuvre must be carried out and repeated if necessary. Antibiotic cover and oxygen should also be given.

Aspiration Pneumonitis. This unfortunately still occurs despite the many precautions taken to prevent it. It is seen in patients who vomit or regurgitate while their cough reflexes are diminished or absent from illness, soporific drugs, or anaesthesia. There are three main occasions when it may occur. The first is under anaesthesia without use of a cuffed endotracheal tube. This has been seen especially in obstetric patients and in them the inhalation of gastric contents of high acidity has produced a gross disturbance of lung function with an asthma-like syndrome—Mendelson's syndrome (Mendelson, 1946). Despite bronchial lavage, corticosteroids, and intermittent positive pressure ventilation (I.P.P.V.), the outlook is grave. The presentation, and detailed management, of these cases have been described by Adams et al (1969). The second occasion is in the immediate post-operative period when recovering from anaesthesia. This was noticed most frequently in acute abdominal emergencies and its incidence was much diminished by the use of naso-gastric tubes. The third occasion is during the course of an illness, or a few days after operation, when vomiting is present due to paralytic ileus. Inhalation of gastric contents at any time is extremely dangerous. The more solid material may produce a granulomatous reaction (Fetterman and Moran, 1942) and the acid juice the Mendelson syndrome mentioned above. If the aspirate is heavily infected, pneumonitis and septic shock may occur.

Treatment. The fluid material should be aspirated immediately. Bronchial lavage with saline or bicarbonate may help in removing it, but, as this is rarely possible to do completely, the beneficial effect is most likely due to dilution or neutralisation of the acid. The further treatment of the pneumonitis or pulmonary oedema is the same as for respiratory failure detailed below.

Pulmonary oedema. This occurs when either the pressure in the pulmonary capillaries is much greater than normal, or the capillaries have leaked out fluid into the pulmonary interstitium. It is thus seen in states of high pulmonary venous pressure such as mitral valve disease or in left ventricular failure. Capillary damage may follow aspiration of irritant fluids or gases or may occur with anaphylactoid states. The symptoms are of respiratory failure, and on auscultation crepitations are heard all over the lungs. The radiological picture is typical.

Treatment. The cause must be treated but it is necessary to improve pulmonary function at once. Where the venous pressure is high, reliance is placed on venesection, digitalis and diuretics. In other causes hydrocortisone may be given in massive doses. A broad spectrum antibiotic should also be given to diminish any associated infection.

Pulmonary Embolism. This is probably increasing although the higher incidence reported may be due to better diagnosis. The embolus originates in the veins of the leg, less often the pelvis. Other sources are from venous anastomosis techniques or suture lines in the venous side of the heart.

Effects of Embolus. There are two main types of pulmonary embolism each produces different signs and symptoms and have a different prognosis.

1. Peripheral Embolism. The embolus may lodge in the distal branches of the pulmonary artery and cause infarction especially when the pulmonary venous pressure is also raised as in mitral stenosis (Braimbridge and Ghadiali, 1965). This produces a reaction in the overlying pleura with roughening and typical pleuritic pain and sometimes a small effusion. Further symptoms of haemoptysis, breathlessness, fever and rapid pulse are typical as is the X-ray picture of a wedge-shaped shadow in the lung periphery. It should, however, be noted that in this, and in acute massive pulmonary embolism, a chest X-ray is frequently unhelpful (Sutton et al, 1969). The peripheral emboli are sometimes multiple and recurrent. They serve as a warning that intensive treatment should be instituted at once before a massive embolus occurs.

2. Massive Central Embolus. This blocks the main pulmonary artery or its branches producing arterial hypotension and central venous hypertension. The rise in venous pressure may be obvious clinically by distension of the neck veins. The clinical picture is one of sudden onset of central chest pain, breathlessness, feeling of apprehension, cyanosis, sweating and collapse. The duration between lodgement of the embolus and death may be a few minutes or a few hours or even days. The story of the patient who on the 8–10th post-operative day sits up in bed, feels the need to defaecate, asks for bedpan and suddenly collapses is familiar to every house-doctor and student. In the surviving patient the differential diagnosis is usually embolism or coronary thrombosis. An X-ray of chest is carried out, but as mentioned before is usually unhelpful as diminished lung vascularity is not always easy to pick up. An E.C.G. is carried out and a central venous line is set up. The E.C.G. may show evidence of right ventricular strain viz. T–wave inversion in the right precordial lead and possibly right bundle branch block. GALLOP rhythm may be present. The central venous line serves to give some idea of the degree of obstruction. A rising C.V.P. is an indication for embolectomy especially if it continues to rise despite treatment. The C.V.P. line also allows pulmonary angiography to be carried out easily, especially if the catheter can be pushed on into the pulmonary artery, and with it assessment of the need for operation. If the main trunks are affected then operation is more likely to be needed. It also allows a follow-up on the effects of therapy. The value of such procedures as angiography, however, must be balanced against the condition of the patient.

Treatment of Pulmonary Embolus

The main line of treatment is conservative with operation reserved for patients who would otherwise die.

Conservative Therapy. The basis of this is anti-coagulation with HEPARIN 10,000 units intravenously every six hours, and an oral anticoagulant PHENINDIONE or WARFARIN. Thrombolytic therapy using Streptokinase or Urokinase has recently become popular but has to be controlled carefully by repeated measurements of various parameters of blood clotting. This therapy has yet to be fully evaluated (McLachlin, 1969). Supportive measures such as oxygen, digitalis, sedatives and vasopressor agents if hypotension is present, are helpful.

Operative Treatment. The problem is one of when to operate. Some apparently moribund patients respond to conservative therapy and live, while others who are apparently well collapse and die.

Broadly speaking surgical intervention should be carried out when there is evidence of insupportable strain on the right ventricle and the risk of death is great. The older technique of pulmonary embolectomy (Trendelenburg, 1908) has been replaced by the use of cardio-pulmonary bypass as in heart operations. Using this the results have improved so that a 50% survival rate has been reported by Paneth (1967), who gives the following indications for operation.

1. One or more episodes of cardiac arrest.
2. A systemic blood-pressure at, or below, 100 mmHg.
3. Tachypnoea, associated with arterial desaturation.
4. Repeated major embolism.

As cardiopulmonary bypass is not, however, available everywhere, there has been a reawakening of interest in the Trendelenburg procedure. Using this in a modified way Clark (1970), of Birmingham has had a 50% survival in desperate cases.

Repeated embolism, especially on anticoagulation, may be treated by ligation or plication of the Inferior Vena Cava. If one is sure by venography, ^{125}I labelled fibrinogen, or ultra sound tests, that the clots originate from the veins of one leg then the superficial femoral vein on the appropriate side only may be ligated.

Respiratory Failure

In defining failure of an organ one usually uses a change in some index of its function as a measure. The obvious index in respiratory failure is that of the blood gas tension. A PCO_2 above 50 mmHg with a PO_2 below 60 mmHg is evidence of failure which may be due to numerous causes: from the respiratory centre controlling respiration: the chest wall incorporating the lungs; to disorder of the lungs themselves. In regard to aetiology, diagnosis, prognosis, and treatment there is a reasonable analogy with disease of other organs in that all these are very much influenced by previous trouble. A disorder which develops in an otherwise healthy lung is much easier to deal with post-operatively than that in one damaged by previous disease. In a series of 80 patients with acute respiratory failure over 70 years of age the mortality rate was 28% (McNicol, 1967). He also emphasised the point that the biochemical severity of the illness in the untreated patient did not influence prognosis.

Treatment. The two main aims in this are to control infection and to relieve hypoxaemia. The principles underlying these should be discussed further.

Control of Infection

The important organisms in the post-operative patient are the Staphylococci, E. Coli, and Ps. Pyocyaneus. These are challenged by various antibiotics depending on their sensitivity which may vary from hospital to hospital. Sputum should be cultured to assess this sensitivity and if possible antibiotic therapy should be withheld until the results are known. There are, however, occasions when a delay may be dangerous. In these cases the antibiotics used must be based on experience and an intelligent guess as to the probable infecting organism. If staphylococci then Benzyl-penicillin (G) pre-operatively is a good first choice with Cloxacillin for the hospital penicillinase resistant organism. Cephaloridine or Chloramphenicol are good alternatives. These are also good for E. Coli, being broad-spectrum antibiotics, and to these may be added Ampicillin, or possibly the combination sulpha methoxazole with Trimethoprin. For pyocyaneus, there are at present three antibiotics whose use should be restricted as resistance may occur. These are Gentamycin and Carbenicillin and Colistin (polymyxin). Carbenicillin is painful when given intramuscularly and should be given in combination with a local anaesthetic agent.

The use of antibiotics does not mean that all efforts to encourage coughing and drainage, and to allow free respiratory movement, should not continue. The usual upright position in bed is not particularly good for allowing drainage of lung bases although breathing is often easier. Post-operative physiotherapy is valuable when the cough is productive but should not be prosecuted too vigorously in the pneumonitis stage.

Control of Hypoxaemia

To do so we must administer the air usually enriched with oxygen in such a way that they reach the alveoli and cross over the alveolar membrane into the blood.

Oxygen Administration

This is usually given by mask to the post-operative patient in concentrations of 30% oxygen or below. It may also be given by endotracheal tube or tracheostomy in patients on a ventilator, where again the concentration should be kept as low as will maintain a satisfactory PO_2. There are, however, times when such a low concentration will not raise a falling PO_2 and higher and higher concentrations are used—not without danger to the patient.

The dangers of oxygen therapy have recently been emphasised in a report for the Scottish Home and Health Department (HMSO, 1969).

Apart from the physical danger of explosion they point out four physiological dangers:

1. Ventilatory Depression. This occurs in patients with a chronically high PCO_2 in whom the respiratory centres response to CO_2 is impaired and who depend on oxygen lack for their respiratory drive. If oxygen lack is removed too quickly respiration will be depressed and the PCO_2 will rise even higher. Only 30% oxygen or less should be used and carefully controlled.

2. Damage to Pulmonary Epithelium. Prolonged inhalation of oxygen at high concentration (60%) can damage pulmonary epithelium (Lorrain–Smith effect), possibly be inactivating surfactant or by a direct effort on the endothelium of the capillaries. Oxygen at 100% takes even less time to produce damage.

3. Oxygen Poisoning. This is seen in diving and in therapy with hyperbaric oxygen and only occurs with high pressures of oxygen. Damage to the C.N.S. may result in convulsions.

4. Retrolental Fibroplasia. This used to occur in babies with administration of oxygen at high concentration. It practically disappeared when concentration was dropped to 40%. Its possibility should still be remembered in the treatment of hyaline membrane disease.

In assessing when to give oxygen to a patient one usually relies on the rather unreliable clinical criteria such as dyspnoea and cyanosis, or in circulatory collapse as in cardiogenic shock. Measurement of PO_2 would be more objective. Eldridge (1966) showed that tissue hypoxia did not occur even at very low oxygen tensions unless hypotension was also present. McNicol (1967) states that oxygen should be given in sufficient concentrations to raise the arterial PO_2 above the assumed safe level (30 mmHg)—a return to normal levels is not necessary. A higher level (50 mmHg) would probably be preferable if any degree of hypotension is present and in the presence of anaemia or known coronary artery disease.

Method of Oxygen Administration

The usual methods are by face mask of which there are various types and by mechanical ventilators. Nasal catheters which project into the anterior nares are satisfactory for controlled oxygen therapy. The various masks have been found useful for delivering oxygen at moderately raised concentrations (Edinburgh and Venturimask) and at high concentration (Polymask or the M.C. mask).

Ventilators

The use of mechanical ventilators should usually be left in the hands of the anaesthetists. Ventilators produce adequate ventilation and oxygenation without effort by the patient. The problems engendered by their use are those of infection, tracheal encrustation and damage, and mechanical damage to the alveoli if they are used improperly. Good humidification will minimise the damage, especially encrustation. The use of ventilators requires the highest standards of care, with tracheal toilet and bronchial aspiration. The nursing care must be excellent and the supervision constant. The patients may require muscle relaxation initially, plus sedation and frequent chest X-ray and blood gas analysis.

It is difficult to know when to begin to take the patient off the ventilator, and, it can be just as difficult to wean them off it. If the arterial PO_2 is 40 mmHg or more breathing room air, the patient should be able to discontinue continual ventilation. He should be allowed off the ventilator for 5 minutes every hour for the first day gradually increasing the interval as his general condition and PO_2 allow. It may take a few days to a week or two for final weaning.

REFERENCES

Adams, A. P., Morgan, M., Jones, B. C. and McCormick, P. W. (1969). A case of massive aspiration of gastric contents during obstetric anaesthesia. *Brit. J. Anaesth.* **41**, 176.

Anscombe, A. R. (1957). Pulmonary Complications of Abdominal Surgery. Lloyd-Luke, Ltd., London.

Braimbridge, M. V. and Ghadiali, P. E. (1965). Post operative cardiac care. Blackwell, Oxford.

Clarke, D. B. (1970). Pulmonary embolectomy. Personal communication.

Comroe, J. H., Forster, R. E., Dubois, A. B., Briscoe, W. A. and Carlsen, E. (1962). The Lung. Clinical physiology and pulmonary function tests. Year Book Medical Publishers Inc., Chicago.

Eldridge, F. (1966). Blood lactate and pyruvate in pulmonary insufficiency. *New Eng. J. Med.* **274,** 878.

Fetterman, G. H. and Moran, T. J. (1942). Food aspiration pneumonia. *Penn. med. J.* **45,** 810.

McIntyre, J. P. (1969). Hypoxia. *Brit. J. Hosp. Med.* **3,** 1113.

McNicol, M. W. (1967). The management of respiratory failure. *Hosp. Med.* **1,** 601.

McLachlin, A. D. (1969). Venous thrombosis and pulmonary embolism. Recent advances in Surgery. Ed. S. Taylor. J. & A. Churchill, Ltd., London.

Mendelson, C. L. (1946). The aspiration of stomach contents into the lungs during obstetric anaesthesia. *Amer. J. Obstet. Gynae.* **52,** 191.

Paneth, M. (1967). The treatment of pulmonary embolism. *Brit. J. Surg.* **54,** 468.

Nunn, J. F. (1970). Applied respiratory physiology. Butterworths, London.

Sutton, G. C., Honey, M. and Gibson, R. A. (1969). Clinical diagnosis of acute massive pulmonary embolism. *Lancet* **1,** 271.

Trendelenburg, F., (1908). Uber die Operative Behandlung der Embolie der Lungenarterie. *Asch. Klin. Cher.* **86,** 686.

Uses and dangers of oxygen therapy. Report of Medical Advisory Committee. H.M.S.O. 1969.

West, J. B. (1965). Ventilation: Blood Flow and Gas Exchange. Blackwell Scientific Publications, Oxford and Edinburgh.

Wright, B. M. and McKerrow, C. B. (1959). *Brit. Med. J.* **2,** 1041.

9: Renal System

As the kidney is the main excretory organ of the body its importance to normal body function is self-evident. Surgery or trauma to the tissues places a strain on renal function, and, if this is already faulty or if the trauma is accompanied by hypotension, sepsis, or excessive tissue breakdown, gross impairment of renal function may result with death of the patient or an increased morbidity.

Much has been learned in recent years on how to prevent renal problems and to sustain or even replace renal function until either the kidneys recover, or suitable alternatives are provided to maintain or take over its excretory function.

Preoperative Assessment of Renal Function

A forewarning of possible renal problems may be given by a history of past renal disease such as glomerulonephritis or pyelonephritis. If not, a history of haematuria or haemoglobinuria, recurrent urinary infections, pyelitis of pregnancy, renal calculi or prostatism should make one suspicious. The presence of hypertension or anaemia should reinforce the suspicion which can be confirmed by tests of renal function.

Tests of Renal Function

There are many elaborate tests of renal function which can utilise biochemical and isotopic laboratories. Information can however be gained in much simpler ways.

Urinalysis

Urine Volume. This is normally about 1,500 ml/day in the adult. An oliguria (400 ml/day) may be due to dehydration or as a part of the normal post-operative response to operation. Complete anuria suggests an obstructive nephropathy or cortical necrosis of the kidney.

Specific Gravity. This relates to the solute load per unit of water. Normally it is about 1,020. It is high with high solute loads and in dehydration and is low in the presence of overhydration or renal failure.

Sediment. In normal patients none should be present or at the most an amorphous non-specific sediment may be seen with a few cells. In dehydration there may be moderate numbers of hyaline and finely granular casts. In renal failure due to acute tubular necrosis there are many tubular cell casts and coarsely granular casts. Red cell and haemoglobin casts may also appear where intravascular haemolysis is present. In obstructive renal disease there may be a scanty sediment and a few red and white cells may be seen with hyaline and finely granular casts.

Electrolytes

In the past a fall in urinary sodium concentration to less than 15 mEq/L was thought to suggest failure of renal function. Normally the urinary sodium concentration is about 40–60 mEq/L but after trauma itself the levels fall dramatically to very low levels of 5–10 mEq/L without deterioration of renal function. Urinary sodium concentrations are therefore of little value.

Urea

About 30–40 g of urea are excreted per day in the urine at a concentration of 2–3 g/100 ml of urine. If the urine volume is low due to dehydration the urea concentration should be high. In renal failure the urea concentration falls to less than 1 g/100 ml so that azotaemia occurs.

The ability of the kidney to remove urea from the blood is used as a measure of its function and as an indication of the glomerular filtration rate (G.F.R.). An average value is 75 ml of blood cleared of urea per minute.

Creatinine

This is another constituent of the urine which may provide information of renal function. It is normally filtered by the glomeruli and excreted at a constant rate. Creatinine clearance may therefore be used as a measure of G.F.R. with only single determinations of blood and urine concentrations required in a 24 hour sample.

Summary. In clinical practice the two measures most commonly used to assess renal function before operation are the blood urea or non-protein nitrogen (remembering the effects of extra-renal factors on this) and the intravenous pyelogram (I.V.P.).

The more elaborate tests of G.F.R., renal plasma flow and tubular function are difficult for routine use and require special techniques. They are probably best left in the hands of the renal physiologist.

Post-operative Assessment of Renal Function

The differentiation of the effects of trauma plus dehydration from true renal failure is an oft recurring problem for the surgeon. A fall in urine output and a rising blood urea certainly makes the distinction essential as the treatment of each is different. The salient features are shown in Fig. 33. To say the least the problem is not always an easy one. Severe hypercatabolic states and factors such as shock, sepsis, and internal and external fluid shifts may obscure the picture. This will be further discussed in the assessment of acute renal failure.

Renal Failure

Definition of this is not as easy as might be thought at first. Such is the reserve of function present that the passage from normal to renal failure is a broad one.

Under normal circumstances the kidneys excrete about 1,500 ml/day. Of this only about 500 ml is necessary to remove the solute load (volume obligatoire)—the rest is free or unattached water. If some degree of renal damage is present or if the solute load is raised e.g. in the hypercatabolic state, then the volume obligatoire rises also, so that in severe chronic renal failure large volumes of dilute urine will be excreted. When the volume of urine excreted is less than can remove the solute load, retention of solutes in the body occurs and renal failure is present.

Acute renal failure is usually due to tubular dysfunction—acute tubular necrosis, and is seen in a variety of surgical conditions where hypotension is accompanied by circulating nephrotoxic substances such as muscle, blood, or bile pigments and endotoxins. It is therefore to be feared in major crushing injuries, resection of ruptured aortic aneurysms, operations on jaundiced patients, open-heart surgery with cardio-pulmonary bypass and operations associated with sepsis especially intraperitoneal infection. This is especially so where the renal function was failing beforehand.

Another even more desperate cause of acute renal failure is acute cortical necrosis. It is fortunately rarely seen in general surgical wards but does occur in obstetric departments. In this condition the cortical glomeruli are destroyed and death is practically invariable as insufficient glomeruli are left to sustain life. If life can be preserved long enough transplant surgery may offer a slim chance of life.

The essential cause of acute tubular necrosis is anoxia of the renal tubules in the presence of the nephrotoxic agents already mentioned. Recovery is possible if diagnosis is made early and essential treatment is instituted.

Diagnosis of Acute Renal Failure

This is based on (a) Oliguria and (b) biochemical evidence of renal damage.

(a) *Oliguria.* As already mentioned it is the low urinary output that alerts the clinician to the possibility of renal damage. Outputs as low as 400 ml/day require active investigation. It must be due to one of three causes—dehydration, renal failure, or to low renal plasma flow—hypotension. The latter is easily corrected by transfusion leaving the other two possibilities. The essential differences between these have already been detailed, Table 29. In problem patients it is common to insert a catheter into the bladder and measure the hourly urine output. This in adults should be above 40 ml/min preferably above 60 ml/min when on intravenous infusions.

Table 29.
POST-OPERATIVE OLIGURIA
Differential Diagnosis

Urine		Dehydration	Acute renal failure
URINE			
Volume		>400 ml/day	<400 ml/day
S.G.		>1·020	<1·015
Sediment		Hyaline & Finely Granular Casts	Tubular Casts
Urea concentration		>1·5 g/100 ml	<1·0 g/100 ml
Electrolytes		Na >40 mEq/l	<15 mEq/l
BLOOD			
P.C.V.		Raised	Low
Urea		Raised	High and Rising
Potassium		Normal	Raised
pH		Normal	Acidosis
RATIOS			
Urea	Urine Blood	>20:1	<14:1
Osmolality	Urine Plasma	>2.5	<1.5
THERAPEUTIC RESPONSE			
I.V. Dextrose		>40 ml/hour	<40 ml/hour

(b) Biochemical Evidence
1. Blood Urea

The normal blood urea of 20–40 mg/100 ml represents a balance between urea production (nitrogen metabolism) and excretion by the kidneys. If the nitrogen load is increased acutely, as for example where massive tissue destruction is present or where blood is present in an extravascular position (gut, tissues, pleural or peritoneal cavities), the blood urea will rise—hypercatabolic response. Another frequent non-renal cause of a raised blood urea is dehydration.

As is well known the blood urea rises following operation. Re-investigating this Bates et al (1970) found a rise, on average, to 48 mgm/100 ml in the first 24 hours after operation. They found also that patients whose blood urea rose by more than 45 mgm/100 ml over the pre-operative level developed renal failure. They emphasised as Porter and Starr (1969) had done that it was the degree of rise in the first 24 hours that was important rather than the total level.

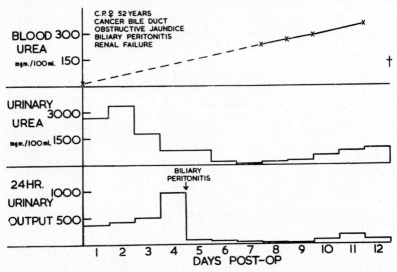

FIG. 33. Renal failure—Urea in urine.

As already mentioned the urinary urea level may also be helpful. A urinary urea concentration of less than 1,100 mgm/100 ml in a pooled specimen was suggested by Molloy (1965) to indicate early renal failure. This may be seen with an "adequate" urine output (Fig. 33).

Various ratios have been used to help further in determining the presence of renal failure such as the urine/plasma osmolality, urine/blood urea, and a refinement of this the "renal excretory index"—

$$\left(\frac{\text{urine urea}}{\text{blood urea}} \times \frac{\text{urine volume}}{100} \right)$$

The normal urine solute excretion is about 1,200 mosmols per 24 hours with a normal urine osmolality of 800–1,000 mosmol/L. Using the average figure of 800 mosmol/L the urine/plasma ratio is approximately 2·5 $\left(\frac{800}{320} \right)$. In dehydration with a high solute low water excretion the ratio will be greater than 2·5 whereas in renal failure the ratio will fall to 1·5 or even less.

The normal blood urea of 20–40 mgm/100 ml contrasts with the urinary urea concentration of approximately 1,300 mgm/100 ml. This gives a urine/blood urea ratio of 40:1 $\left(\frac{1300}{30} \right)$. Where this ratio is

increased it means an increased solute load with a steady blood urea
or a fall in blood urea or a balance of the two as they rise together but
with an increase in favour of the solute load per unit of blood or total

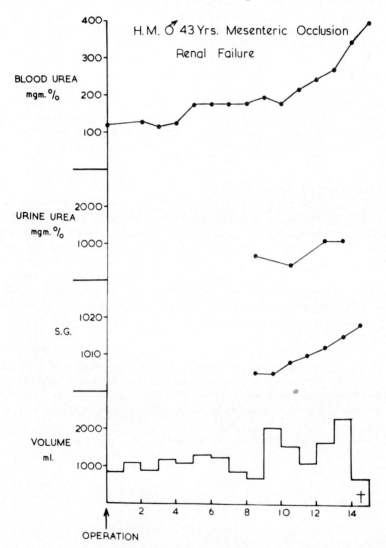

FIG. 34. Renal failure plus a hypercatabolic state.

body water i.e. as occurs in dehydration. A fall in the ratio to below
14:1 occurs early in renal failure (Perlmutter, Crossman, Rothenburg
and Dobkin, 1959). Later this ratio can drop below 5:1. At low ratios
the chances of survival are small. The refinement of this ratio was

introduced by Lindsay, Linton and Longland (1965) who considered the total 24 hour urine output. They claimed that a renal excretory index of less than 84 was indicative of acute renal failure. A problem of using 24 hour urine collections is the need for catheterisation of the bladder, but, despite the fear of infection, it is often done. False positives have been observed in studies using these ratios but perhaps this is not a bad thing as it is better to be alerted more often than is necessary.

In view of the complexity of some of these ratios it is comforting that Bates, Pigott and Stableforth found that the degree in rise in blood urea in the first 24 hours was as good an indication of acute renal failure as any. They recognised, as has already been stressed, that the differentiation of pre-renal from renal failure cannot always be clear cut.

Treatment of Renal Failure

As recovery from acute tubular necrosis is possible, treatment is aimed at correcting haemodynamic, bacteriological and metabolic problems already present, and sustaining the body long enough for regeneration of the tubular epithelium. The problem is rarely straight-forward especially in surgical cases as added to the above problems are those consequent upon operations on tissues. Often the patients suffer from incidental disease such as atherosclerosis, diabetes, respiratory disease, etc. It is necessary therefore to plan the treatment for the individual and his problem bearing in mind some principles common to most, if not all.

In any given case a simple suitable programme may be outlined:—

1. General examination for signs of dehydration, fluid shifts, blood loss and infection. The blood pressure is checked and a chest X-ray and E.C.G. is carried out.

2. Pass a urethral catheter for hourly urine output (despite risk of infection).

3. An intragastric tube may be necessary.

4. Remove blood for full blood count, blood culture and biochemical analysis.

This includes urea, creatinine, electrolytes, osmolality and acid-base parameters. Crossmatching of blood should be done if anaemia is present.

5. Urinalysis—specific gravity, pH, sediment, culture, electrolytes, urea, creatinine and osmolality.

From the above the differential diagnosis should usually be possible (refer Table 29). If not then one must start with correction of deficits and tests of cure.

Correction of Deficits:—

1. Correct fluid and electrolyte disturbances.

2. Treat sepsis if present. Note some antibiotics, e.g. Kanamycin are nephrotoxic.
3. If anaemia present may need blood transfusion. But note haemolysis could lead to further damage.
4. Excise devitalised tissue, crushed muscle, gangrenous limbs, etc.

Tests of Cure

1. Intravenous fluids. A litre of saline or, if plasma sodium is above normal, 5% glucose is given rapidly over an hour. If the urine output increases to more than 40 ml/hour then renal failure is not present and the dehydration state can be treated. If there is no result Mannitol can be tried.

2. Mannitol. This promotes a diuresis by raising the osmolality of the urine. It should be used with care however as it can produce pulmonary oedema if not excreted and like most diuretics removes electrolytes with the water. Usually some 50 ml of a 25% solution of Mannitol is given over 5 minutes. The urinary output should rise to more than 40 ml/hour during the next 3 hours. If not, a further 100 ml of 25% solution can be given over 10 minutes or divided into two 50 ml doses at three hourly intervals. If diuresis does not occur then acute renal failure is presumed. If a response is obtained then a further litre of 10% Mannitol plus fluid and electrolytes for further maintenance may be given over the next 24 hours.

3. Diuretics. Large doses of FRUSEMIDE may be used if one is reasonably sure that severe dehydration is not present. An intravenous dose of 40 mg may be given and repeated in 6 to 8 hours. If there is no response then renal failure is likely to be present.

Specific Treatment

There are 3 main principles in treatment.
1. Maintain water and electrolyte balance.
2. Restrict protein breakdown.
3. Treat complications as they arise or attempt to prevent them.

1. Maintenance of water and electrolyte balance

Water comes from 2 sources endogenous and exogenous. The amount which must be given depends on that produced in the body, which in itself is dependent on the metabolic rate and the fluid content of the individual. Normally about 400 ml of water is endogenously produced per day. In catabolism of fat and hypercatabolic state in general it may be higher even up to 1,000 ml/day.

A reasonably acceptable estimate of the amount which should be given to the patient is 400 ml/day. Further amounts depend on fluid losses into gut, sweating, rapid respiration and that passed in the urine.

These are added to the basic figure of 400 ml/day to give the total fluid intake. The electrolyte intake depends on past losses, present losses and plasma levels. It is difficult to estimate past losses. The present losses are those in the urine and can be estimated. The plasma sodium may reflect not a loss but an accumulation of water-sodium dilution. The changes in plasma potassium reflect the rapidity of protein break-down.

If possible it is best to have a weight bed available in the treatment of these patients and aim for a loss in weight of 0·2 Kg/day.

2. *Prevention of protein breakdown*

A certain amount of this must occur as part of the metabolic response to a stressful situation. It can be limited to some extent by maintaining water balance and supplying calories especially in the form of glucose. If protein breakdown can be halved, then the rate at which the blood urea rises will be about 20 mg/100 ml, and that of potassium by the order of 0·3 mEq/L/day.

The calorie need of a patient varies from 1,000–4,000 cals/day depending on the state of catabolism. It is difficult to give this by mouth with the amount of fluid available. High calorie oral preparations which are protein free have been produced, e.g. HYCAL (Beecham Laboratories) which can provide 425 cals in 175 ml of fluid. This preparation is somewhat nauseating, only less so if soda water is added. Hypertonic glucose, or perhaps better fructose, is given by a cannula in the inferior vena cava or intravenous fat may be used. In time, such is the protein breakdown, that some exogenous protein is required usually in combination with fructose and ethanol. Finally, vitamins will need to be given with the fluid-supplements.

3. *Complications*

In acute failure the main ones are overhydration, hyperkalaemia, renal acidosis, infection and anaemia. The treatment of these is dealt with in appropriate chapters. Anaemia in renal disease is common, and, as transfusion problems are great, a level of 75% haemoglobin is thought to be acceptable.

Renal Dialysis

If conservative measures fail then recourse to some form of renal dialysis will be necessary. With this the mortality has been reduced to about 40–50% (Gallagher and Polak, 1967).

Indications for Dialysis

The commonest indications are a raised serum potassium above 7 mEq/L and a blood urea above 300 mg/100 ml. Added to these are a deteriorating clinical state and in the case of drug poisons, the need to eliminate these.

Methods of dialysis

There are two main methods: peritoneal and haemodialysis. *Peritoneal dialysis* is the more commonly used one is the surgical wards as the equipment required is not sophisticated or expensive and it can be carried out in a non-specialised unit. In simple terms the procedure consists in the insertion of a catheter, specially adapted in the form of a trocar and obturator, into the peritoneal cavity. Local anaesthetic is used and the best site of insertion is in the midline one third of the distance down from the umbilicus to the symphysis pubis. The catheter is used for the instillation of dialysis fluid which is left in the peritoneal cavity for up to an hour and is then siphoned off. The cycle of instillation and removal is repeated a number of times, perhaps 20–30, depending on the needs and the biochemical and clinical response.

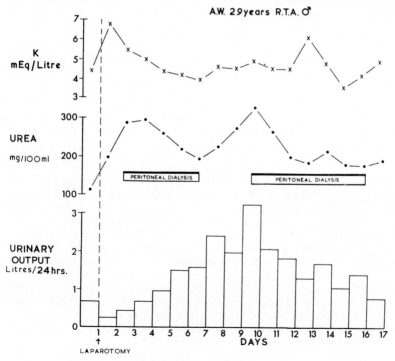

Fig. 35. Peritoneal dialysis.

The results are illustrated of a 29 year old man who was involved in a road traffic accident. He had a laparotomy and splenectomy. Following this he required dialysis twice in treatment of renal failure. He finally recovered.

The technique has obvious dangers which were fully discussed by Ledingham (1970). An example of its value is shown in Fig. 35.

Haemodialysis

Artificial kidney machines are described as rapid or slow according to their size and the rapidity with which they change the urea and electrolytes. A too rapid change in urea can set up a problem in osmotic gradient with cellular oedema—the dialysis disequilibration syndrome of Kennedy, Linton and Eaton (1962).

Haemodialysis is practically only carried out in a special renal unit. The various techniques used and the relevant suitability of each has been well described by Gallagher and Polak (1967).

Chronic Renal Failure

This presents a serious problem in surgical patients in whom the trauma of operation on an already damaged kidney may produce acute on chronic renal failure.

Suspicion as to the presence of chronic renal disease is usually aroused by the presence of an unexplained normocytic anaemia and is confirmed by finding a high blood urea, which incidentally does not seem to be troubling the patient. Renal calcification and appearance of small renal shadows on plain X-ray and poor function on I.V.P. are all confirmatory of chronic renal disease. Absolute confirmation comes from renal function tests, urinalysis and, if necessary, renal biopsy.

If, after operation, acute on chronic renal failure does develop, it will probably be necessary to insert an arterio venous shunt and prepare for haemodialysis. It is better to be early in the treatment of this most serious and sometimes intractable problem.

REFERENCES

Bates, C. P., Pigott, H. W. S. and Stableforth, P. G. (1970). Changes in blood-urea concentrations after operations and their relation to the early diagnosis of acute renal failure. *Brit. J. Surg.* **57**, 360.

Porter, G. A. and Starr, A. (1969). Management of post-operative renal failure following cardiovascular surgery. *Surgery*, St. Louis **65**, 390.

Molloy, P. J. (1962). The early diagnosis of impaired post-operative renal function. *Lancet* **2**, 696.

Perlmutter, M., Grossman, S. L., Rothenberg, S. and Dobkin, G. (1959). Urine-serum urea nitrogen ratio; simple test of renal function in acute azotemia and oliguria. *J.A.M. Med. Ass.* **170**, 1533.

Lindsay, R. M., Linton, A. L. L. and Longland, C. J. (1965). Assessment of Postoperative renal function. *Lancet* **1**, 978.

Gallagher, L. and Polak, A. (1967). The management of acute renal failure. *Hosp. Med.* **1**, 287.

Kennedy, A. C., Linton, A. L. and Eaton, J. C. (1962). Urea levels in cerebrospinal fluid after dialysis. *Lancet* **1**, 410.

Ledingham, J. (1970). Peritoneal dialysis. *Brit. J. Hospital Medicine*, **4**, 85.

10: Liver

Surgical interest in the liver has, until recently, been focussed on the treatment of surgical jaundice, the control of portal hypertension, local resection for tumours and the repair of lacerations. An improved understanding of the surgical anatomy of the liver and the principles of intensive care has encouraged more venturesome procedures, culminating in total liver replacement. The operations are designed on anatomical principles and are governed by a knowledge of liver physiology. With these and immunosuppression, the future looks brighter in liver surgery. Some of the principles will be discussed further.

It is impossible to give a brief summary of the physiology of an organ which has over 500 known functions. All are important to the normal body metabolism. Only a few have direct relevance to surgery. These will be discussed and the applied anatomy in relation to resection summarised.

Anatomical Consideration and Partial Resection

The liver appears to be divided by the falciform ligament into right and left lobes. But, as Cantlie (1898) pointed out, this is a superficial impression (Fig. 36). The dividing line is actually about 3 cm to the right falciform ligament in the line of the inferior vena cava marked inferiorly by the gall-bladder fossa. To the left of this main lobar fissure is the left lobe which is divided into medial and lateral segments by the left segmental fissure, which corresponds to the line of attachment of the falciform ligament. The lateral segment is the classic left lobe of the liver; the medial segment includes the quadrate and most of the caudate lobes.

The right lobe is divided further into anterior and posterior segments by another fissure which extends downwards from the junction of the superior and posterior surfaces in an anterior direction. These, and other fissures, were described by Hjortsjö (1963) and their importance in liver surgery was beautifully detailed by Bengmark (1968). The fissures are relatively vascular areas in which run the hepatic radicals.

Partial resection has become the treatment of choice for severe crushing injuries to the liver as well as for primary and some solitary secondary neoplasms. Resection is carried out in the emergency case with the assistant compressing the liver between his thumbs and fingers on sectioning the tissue, either using the finger method of Lin et al (1960) or the handle of a scalpel (Quattlebaum, 1953). In non-emergency situations, a formal dissection of the portal hepatis is carried out. The results of resection are excellent if done early after injury. Where less than 10 units of blood were used 8 out of 9 patients survived whereas when over 10 units of blood were used, there was only one survival in 10 patients (Perry, 1970).

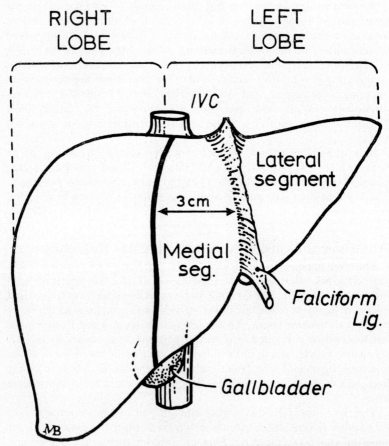

FIG. 36. Surface anatomy of the liver.

Major resections of liver tissue, especially if carried out as an emergency procedure, may be followed by hepatic and/or renal failure. In the planned operation, these complications are less likely. Some degree of liver dysfunction usually follows surgery on the liver. The serum bilirubin rises quickly and parallels the amount resected. In major resections it may take a few weeks to return to normal. If the common bile duct is drained at operation, the degree of rise is reduced. The most important metabolic change is a fall in serum albumin (Chapter 3). For this reason, repeated infusions of albumin and plasma are necessary post-operatively. The disturbance in protein metabolism is also indicated by a fall in blood urea. The blood coagulation factors may also be affected by operation, but a specific bleeding tendency is not common, especially when Vitamin K is given. The risk of a hepatic encephalopathy is diminished by giving an intestinal antibiotic such as neomycin preoperatively if possible.

Infusion Therapy in Malignant Disease

The fact that primary and secondary tumours of the liver derive most of their blood supply from the hepatic artery, has led to the intra-arterial infusion of chemotherapeutic agents in the treatment of these. The catheter is inserted at operation or by retrograde passage via the femoral or brachial arteries. Recent reports have shown the benefit of intra-arterial 5-fluorouracil in treatment of hepatomas (Provan et al, 1968), and secondary tumours (Murray–Lyon et al, 1970). The latter authors showed that liver function was moderately disturbed but none of their patients developed liver failure. Apart from infusion, hepatic artery ligation, suggested by Markousitz (1952), has been tried with some success either alone or following infusion. Although the early attempts at ligation of the hepatic artery were followed by a high mortality (Graham and Cannel, 1933), the later studies demonstrated that when hypotension and sepsis were avoided there was very little disturbance of liver function (Almersjö et al, 1967). Hepatic artery ligation followed by infusion of drugs through the portal vein has been also carried out with some success. These procedures should be accompanied by infusion of fructose for metabolic support within the liver.

Obstructive Jaundice

This usually refers to jaundice due to stone or malignant disease which may be relieved by surgery. The 3 main hazards of surgery in obstructive jaundice are, haemorrhage, liver failure, and the hepato-renal syndrome.

The bleeding tendency is due to failure of absorption of Vitamin K from the gut because of absence of bile salts. The prothrombin level in the blood falls, and must be raised before operations. In an emergency situation, the prothrombin level can be raised by the intravenous injection of 20 mg Menadione (Vit. K1) which can be repeated in 2–3 hours. Its success can be checked by estimation of prothrombin activity. Fresh, frozen or dried plasma may also be used, as the prothrombin in it remains active for several months. In the non-emergency situation, Vitamin K can be given daily by intramuscular injection.

Liver failure after surgery on an obstructed biliary system is less common now, as surgeons are more ready to carry out laparotomy early, before the liver function suffers from unremitting obstruction. It is important to protect the liver as far as possible during and after operation by; intravenous fructose, antibiotics, and by maintaining a stable blood pressure and blood volume.

The hepato-renal syndrome is an extension of the above, where renal failure and hepatic failure co-exist. This complication has also been largely eliminated by paying attention to pre- and post-operative diuresis by infusion of 10% Mannitol, as well as the control of infection and changes in blood pressure.

Hepatic Encephalopathy

Neuropsychiatric disturbances (hepatic encephalopathy) have been observed in patients with liver disease for a long time. It is due to the effect on the brain of a toxic substance or substances which come from the gut via the portal vein and which are not detoxicated by the liver. The failure of detoxication is due either to parenchymatous liver disease (cirrhosis) or to a shunting of the blood past the liver or usually a combination of these. There are two types of shunts which bypass the liver: the normal porto-systemic collateral circulation which opens up when portal flow through the liver is hindered and the surgical shunt or porto-caval anastomosis.

The exact nature of the toxic substances which affect the brain is not fully known. They would appear to be derived from nitrogenous compounds and, although not alone, ammonia (NH_3) is implicated. This is further discussed below. The factors responsible for hepatic encephalopathy are illustrated in Fig. 37. They start with the breakdown of nitrogenous compounds (blood and protein) in the gut, by bacteria, into NH_3 and other possible toxic substances. These pass up the portal vein to the liver where they should be detoxicated. If the liver fails to detoxify the material or if porto-systemic shunts (normal or man-made) are large enough, the toxic agents pass to the brain. Even there, some protection is afforded by youth as the encephalopathy is commoner in the older person.

Clinically, the condition may be acute, especially in the post-operative cases, or chronic as in the long standing cirrhotics, or developing months after shunt operations. It is said to occur in about 20% of cases following porto-caval anastomosis (Sherlock, 1967), with an incidence of just over 10% with end to side porto-caval anastomosis and about 30% with side to side anastomosis. The clinical features vary from drowsiness, inattention, trouble with co-ordination, brisk reflexes, foetid breath, flapping tremor to coma. The diagnosis is made clinically with support from an E.E.G. and blood ammonia levels.

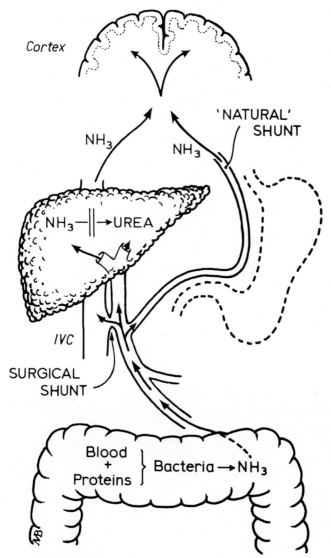

FIG. 37. Mechanisms of hepatic encephalopathy.

Prevention

In surgical practice, hepatic encephalopathy is most commonly seen after operations for the control of bleeding from oesophageal varices.

The large amount of protein in the gut after a haemorrhage provides a ready source of toxic agents. Add to this, the effect of anaesthesia, trauma, hypotension and possibly infection on liver cell function. Potassium depletion may also be present due to previous diuretics and is thought to precipitate hepatic coma by increasing the ammonia production by the kidney (Baertl et al, 1963). To avoid the problem, the various factors responsible should be eliminated. The bowel should be cleansed of blood, and hypotension, etc., should be prevented. Porto-caval anastomosis should be performed only where the liver function is satisfactory as denoted by a serum albumin level of more than 3 g/100 ml. As the risk of encephalopathy increases with age, it is best to operate on those below the age of 50 years and who are not suffering from jaundice or ascites.

It is suggested that in patients who have had porto-caval anastomosis an E.E.G. should be carried out at regular intervals to detect the signs of slowing which signify an early reversible preclinical stage (Read et al, 1968 and Hawkes et al, 1970).

Treatment

The main principles in the management of hepatic encephalopathy are the same for all, but differ, of course, in the intensity of application according to the degree of neurological disturbance present. They are:—

1. Elimination of nitrogenous substances from the gut.

In the acute case, this will require twice daily bowel washouts to get rid of the blood. In the milder case, protein is eliminated from the diet.

2. Suppression of bacterial action in the gut.

This is carried out in 2 ways. First, by the use of antibiotics such as Neomycin, given initially orally as 2 g every 6 hours reducing to 1 g 6 hourly. The second, and ancillary method, is to give lactulose (50 g per day) a synthetic disaccharide. This sugar reaches the terminal ileum and colon unchanged, and there it favours the growth of saccharolytic organisms at the expense of the proteolytic ones. The lactulose is broken down by bacterial fermentation to lactic acid and small amounts of other acids, thus dropping the faecal pH to 4·5–5·5. There is a decrease in the formation of ammonia (NH_3) ions and increase in the nonabsorbable ammonium (NH_4) ions (Rud, 1970).

3. Support liver functions and correct electrolyte changes.

The first is achieved by an adequate calorie intake, usually in the form of hypertonic dextrose or fructose into a catheter in the vena cava. Oral feeding, or feeding by a stomach tube, may be possible in whole or, at least, in part. The electrolyte status should be assessed.

As these patients usually hold on to sodium, only limited amounts are necessary intravenously. A low potassium state should be corrected.

4. Surgical treatment.

Surgery is perhaps best reserved for the more chronic relapsing forms of encephalopathy and aims to remove the source of NH_3 where its production cannot be controlled by more conservative means. The various methods used have been; total colectomy, ileostomy and ileo-sigmoid anastomosis. The results of these have so far proved to be of value but long-term assessment is necessary to define their role.

Ammonia (NH_3)

This is produced in the lower gut by the action of bacteria on protein. It is carried in the portal blood to the liver where it is metabolised through the Krebs cycle to urea. Very little ammonia passes into the general circulation (Fig. 37). Even when an ammonium salt is given by mouth, it is difficult to produce a sustained rise in the blood ammonia levels. In cirrhosis with bypass of the liver, or in porto-caval shunts, elevated ammonia levels may be detected in the blood.

In recent years, there has been improvement in the technique for measuring blood ammonia. The normal level of ammonia in peripheral venous blood is less than 30 μg per 100 ml, with an upper limit of normal of 50 μg per 100 ml (Fenton, 1967). The arterial blood level, which is mostly used in studies is 10 μg per 100 ml higher than in venous blood. In hepatic coma the levels may be raised to above 200 μg per 100 ml. But the blood ammonia level is not always raised even in severe coma. It is often enough, however, to make the diagnosis of hepatic encephalopathy suspect, if the ammonia level is not raised. It is said that an increase in blood ammonia level may precede the onset of symptoms as a fall precedes recovery (Stahl, 1963). There may be substances other than ammonia responsible for the neuropsychiatric disturbances. However, there is little doubt that prevention of raised ammonia levels is important in patients with poor liver function. Every effort must be made clinically to keep the blood ammonia level low by actively removing protein from the gut and diminishing bacterial activity. Enemas, antibiotics, and even haemodialysis to remove ammonia, all play their part.

Liver Failure

This is more difficult to define than renal failure. Disturbances of liver function tests are always found if previous liver disease or acute hepatocellular damage is present. None of these are very precise and they do not have the same significance in relation to the extent and progress of the problem as does the blood urea in renal failure. It must be remembered that in hepatic failure the blood urea falls.

The clinical picture is reasonably clear. Hepatic failure is seen in patients who have cirrhosis with or without portal hypertension, and especially those subjected to operation for bleeding varices, who have had a hepatotoxic anaesthetic agent or other drugs; suffered from toxaemia associated with sepsis; or who have developed severe hepatitis. Rarely, it may be seen in severe shock. The appearance in such patients of neurological symptoms, especially dulling of consciousness going on to coma, of warm hands with a flapping tremor, ascites and spider naevi, and in some cases, an enlarged tender liver should suggest the presence of liver failure. The electrolyte changes vary according to the cause. Patients with cirrhosis retain fluid easily, an excess water and salt develops and the plasma volume expands. They are, therefore, treated with a low sodium diet, diuretics, and an aldosterone antagonist (spironolactone). The tendency to lose potassium is corrected by potassium supplements. The plasma albumin may be low. The essential electrolyte changes are thus, hypokalaemia, hyponatraemia and hypoalbuminaemia. The hypokalaemia is the most important problem and may develop rapidly in patients after liver operations, sometimes in association with alkalosis. Hyponatraemia may be due to dilution in the body water or to diuretic therapy and is then of little significance if the blood pressure is normal. It may, however, in the seriously ill patient reflect the passage of sodium into the cells and may indicate impending death. When the serum sodium falls below 125 mEq/L recovery is rare (Hecker and Sherlock,1956).

Treatment

Patients with liver failure qualify for really intensive care involving management of the renal, cardiac and respiratory problems as has been described. When all else fails, thought must be given to means of extracorporeal hepatic support. This is a relatively new field of which more may be expected in the future.

Extracorporeal Hepatic Support

Before considering the various techniques available, it should be emphasised that patients in hepatic failure differ from those in renal failure, in that many of the conditions producing the problem, are at present, irreversible. This may not always be so and, indeed, further evaluation of hepatic support techniques may make this clearer.

1. Haemodialysis

This has been used in much the same way as in renal failure. At present, the results are much less satisfactory (Keynes, 1968). Exchange transfusions using blood or plasma have also been used, but risks inherent in them and the results, so far, make their value questionable.

They have also been used in support of cross-circulation techniques involving the baboon (Saunders et al, 1968, Terblanche and Bosman, 1968).

2. Heterologous Perfusion

The isolated pig's liver has been used to support organ function. In this, the patient's blood is perfused through the pig liver which may function for about 8 hours. Patients have emerged from coma after perfusion but there are many problems in this technique, which is however capable of further development. Multiple perfusions are often required and the development of antibodies has even led to more than one animal species being used to provide livers for perfusion (Abouna et al, 1970, Kirkley, Hull, Ashcroft and Kerr, 1969).

3. Hepatic Homotransplantation

Much interest has been shown in this, as, like cardiac replacement it would seem to be the logical answer for patients with the irrepairably damaged organs. There are many problems in obtaining suitable livers particularly as the liver is very susceptible to even short periods of warm ischaemia. Rejection and the best methods of tissue typing and the control of rejection have also still to be solved (Calne, 1969). Liver replacement by transplantation is thus a long way behind renal transplantation at the present time.

REFERENCES

Cantlie, J. (1898). On a new arrangement of the right and left lobes of the liver. *Proc. Anat. Soc. Great Britain and Ireland* **32,** 4.

Hjortsjö, C. H. (1963). The anatomical foundations of liver surgery. Proceeding from 2nd World Congress of Gastroenterology Munich **111,** 523.

Bengmark, S. (1968). Liver surgery. Progress in surgery **6.** S. Karger. Basel & New York.

Lin, T. Y., Chen, K. M. and Lin, T. K. (1960). Total right hepatic lobectomy for primary hepatoma. *Surgery* **48,** 1048.

Quattlebaum, J. K. (1953). Massive resection of the liver. *Ann. Surg.* **137,** 787.

Perry, J. F. (1970). Blunt and penetrating abdominal injuries. Current problems in Surgery. May 1970. Year Book Medical Publishers Inc. (Chicago).

Provan, J. L., Stokes, J. F. and Edwards, D. (1968). Hepatic artery infusion chemotherapy in hepatoma. *Brit. med. J.* **2,** 346.

Murray-Lyon, I. M., Dawson, L. J., Parsons, V. A., Rade, M. O., Blendis, L. M. and Laws, J. W. (1970). Treatment of secondary hepatic tumours by ligation of hepatic artery and infusion of cytotoxic drugs. *Lancet* **2,** 172.

Markowitz, J. (1952). The hepatic artery.

Markowitz, J., Rappaport, A., and Scott, A. C. (1949). The function of the hepatic artery in the dog. *Amer. J. digest. Dis.* **16,** 344.

Abouna, G. M., Serron, B., Boehmig, H. G., Amemy, A. H. and Martineau, G. (1970). Longterm hepatic support by intermittent long term liver perfusions. *Lancet* **2,** 391.

Graham, R. R. and Cannel, D. (1933). Accidental legation of the hepatic artery. Report of one case, with a review of the cases in the literature. *Brit. J. Surg.* **20,** 566.

Almersjö, O., Bengmark, S., Engevik, L., Hafstrom, L. O., Loughbridge, B. P. and Nilsson, L. A. V. (1968). Serum enzyme changes after hepatic dearterialisation in man. *Ann. Surg.* **167,** 9.

Sherlock, S. (1967). In The Liver p. 242 (Edited by A. E. Read). London.

Baertl, J. M., Sancetta, S. M. and Gabuzda, G. J. (1963). Relation of acute potassium depletion to renal ammonium metabolism in patients with cirrhosis. *J. Clin. Invest.* **42,** 696.

Read, A. E., McCarthy, C. F., Ajdukiewicz, A. B. and Brown, G. J. A. (1968). Encephalopathy after portacaval anastomosis *Lancet* **2,** 999.

Hawkes, C. H., MacPherson, A. I. S., Pryor, H. and Townsend, H. R. A. (1970). The value of E.E.G. frequency analysis in hepatic encephalopathy *J. Roy. Coll. Surg. Edin.* **15,** 151.

Editorial Lancet (1970). Treatment of chronic hepatic encephalopathy. *Lancet* **2,** 449.

11: Gastrointestinal Metabolic Problems

The daily exchange of fluid and electrolytes between the body and the intestinal lumen is considerable. About 8 litres enters the upper alimentary tract from the intestinal glands and mouth daily yet only about 100 ml are excreted in the faeces (Fig. 38). Fluid and electrolytes are also being transferred constantly to and fro across the intestinal mucosa and any alteration in normal transport through the intestine can cause rapid and extensive losses from the body. Nutritional disturbances are never a problem in the early stages of the management of acute losses.

The extent and nature of the alteration in fluid and electrolyte balance and H$^+$ regulation depends on the composition and volume of the gastroinstestinal fluid which is either lost or sequestrated in a paralysed intestine (Table 30). The special problems associated with

Table 30.

DAILY VOLUMES (ml.) AND IONIC CONCENTRATIONS mEq/L OF GASTROINTESTINAL FLUIDS COMPARED TO PLASMA

	Vol. (ml)	Na+	Cl$^-$	K+	HCO3$^-$	H+
Plasma	3500	140	103	4.0	25	
Gastric	500–2500	50	120	15	20	70
Biliary	700	140	100	15	40	–
Pancreatic	800	160	75	10	80	–
Intestinal	3000	120	110	20	30	–

obstruction and fistulae at various sites will be considered. Obstruction at the duodenojejunal junction produces the greatest deficit in the shortest time. Obstruction at various sites leads to varying patterns of metabolic disorder.

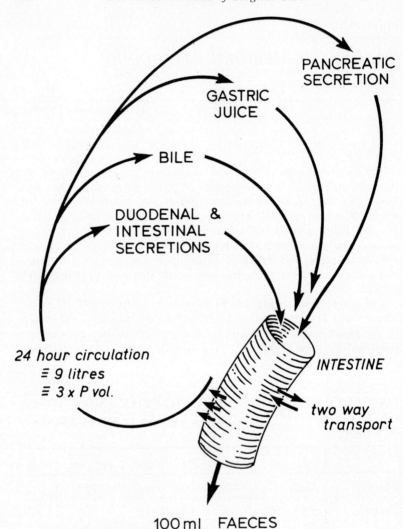

PANCREATIC
SECRETION

GASTRIC
JUICE

BILE

DUODENAL &
INTESTINAL
SECRETIONS

24 hour circulation
   ≡ 9 litres
   ≡ 3 x P vol.

INTESTINE

two way
transport

100 ml   FAECES

FIG. 38. Volume of alimentary secretions in health.

Pyloroduodenal Obstruction

The commonest cause of pyloric stenosis is chronic duodenal ulceration. Stenosis develops slowly and obstruction is seldom complete. Vomiting of gastric secretions and food is replaced usually by drinking hypotonic fluids, some of which will pass the obstruction so that electrolyte and acid base imbalance is greater than in acute small intestinal obstruction where dehydration predominates. Some patients remain remarkably well compensated even after many days of vomiting.

Metabolic Effects

The daily losses become greater as stenosis progresses and the volume of gastric secretion rises in response to prolonged distension and so augments the losses. Disorders of electrolytes and acid base balance are due to loss of cation as hydrogen, and anions as sodium and chloride. The concentration of chloride in gastric secretions is between 100 and 120 mEq per litre and of sodium between 50 and 100 mEq per litre, thus the loss of chloride is correspondingly greater than the loss of sodium. Potassium is also lost in the vomit to the extent of about 20 mEq per litre and an appreciable potassium deficit can develop as vomiting persists.

The loss of H^+ in pyloric obstruction without loss of base leads to an increase in serum pH. Carbonic acid dissociates in the parietal cells into H^+ which passes into the stomach and is lost: HCO_3, on the other hand, enters the extracellular space and the plasma level rises. There is a close relationship between the plasma concentration of chloride and bicarbonate, as the chloride level falls the bicarbonate level rises (Howe and Le Quesne, 1964).

The excess bicarbonate is excreted initially in the urine as a compensating mechanism in association with sodium and potassium. These ions however become further depleted as vomiting continues and when they cease to be available the production of an alkaline urine stops. As vomiting persists and more and more sodium is lost, body fluid tonicity and the maintenance of plasma volume are threatened. Potassium instead of sodium and increasing amounts of H^+ begin to be excreted in the urine and the paradox develops of a patient with alkalosis and hypokalaemia secreting an acid urine. The rising extracellular pH and bicarbonate levels lower the ionised calcium level in blood and tetany may develop.

Clinical Findings

Patients with pyloric stenosis usually have an associated nutritional deficiency and weight loss associated with repeated vomiting over many months. Weight loss is further increased by dehydration. Thirst is present, the mucous membranes become dry. Clinical evidence of sodium depletion is reflected by apathy, sunken eyes and lax subcutaneous tissues. In advanced situations peripheral circulatory failure and hypotension develop. The serum and urine electrolyte levels indicate the severity of the losses which have occurred. The standard bicarbonate levels give a good idea of the alkalotic state and levels of over 40 mEq per litre are often associated with tetany. The extent of the increase of the blood pH is variable and values of 7·50–7·60 are common. The concentration of electrolytes in urine may be deceptively normal. Mild hypokalaemia and hypochloraemia are usually found when serum is examined. The blood urea is raised to 150–180 mg per 100 ml due to the combined water and salt deficit. The urine may still be alkaline in a mild case but later small quantities of an acid and virtually salt

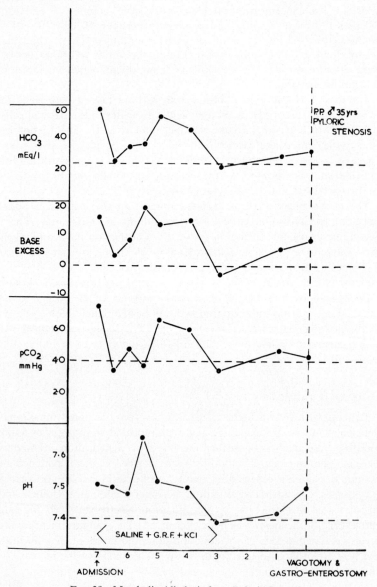

FIG. 39. Metabolic Alkalosis from Pyloric Stenosis.

free urine with an increased specific gravity will be passed. Some of the biochemical findings in a 35 year old patient are shown in Fig. 39.

Treatment

When clinical signs of dehydration are marked, a mixed water and salt deficit amounting to 4 or 5 litres is present. Treatment initially aims to restore the fluid, electrolyte and acid base balance as quickly as possible. Isotonic saline and 5% Dextrose in equal amounts is infused initially. If a sodium deficit remains after twenty four hours then hypertonic saline can be added. Potassium depletion is catered for by adding KCl to the infusion at a rate of about 12–15 mEq K per hour. Surgical correction of the obstruction is planned and two to three days is usually all that is required to prepare the patient for safe surgery.

Small Intestinal Obstruction

Mechanical obstruction at the region of the pyloroduodenal junction causes a very rapid clinical deterioration due to large fluid losses whereas an obstruction of the terminal ileum produces a gradual deterioration as intestinal fluid can be absorbed from proximal loops of small intestine.

The extent of the metabolic changes depends on the site of the obstruction. Paralysis and dilatation of the small intestine in peritonitis or after complicated abdominal surgery establishes a further temporary body fluid compartment which increases in size at the expense of the extracellular fluid space. A decrease in the E.C.F. causes an increase in the packed cell volume which is proportional to the fall in plasma volume. For example a 20% increase in the haematocrit indicates an approximate 30% reduction in plasma volume. In patients who have not lost blood, a packed cell volume of 55% on admission signifies a 30% fall in plasma volume and a deficit of similar proportion in the rest of the extracellular space. The fluid lost is isotonic with plasma and therefore there is little change in the serum electrolyte concentrations in the early stages of small intestinal obstruction or ileus. Low serum sodium levels may indicate the production of sodium free water from endogenous fat metabolism or persistently low sodium intakes during replacement therapy.

Further accumulation of fluid and electrolytes develops in the obstructed segment due to an increased rate of transport of water, sodium and potassium into the lumen of the bowel and a reduced rate of passage in the opposite direction (Shields, 1964).

Some of the factors responsible for this reduced ability to handle fluid and electrolytes are distension and vascular insufficiency with an increased venous pressure in the wall of the bowel.

Acid base imbalance may develop later as small intestinal obstruction persists. The pH and the standard bicarbonate will fall due to an excessive loss of base into the gut. Hypoxia of large segments of intestine as well as starvation ketosis will also lower the pH.

Treatment

The prime consideration in management consists in a clinical assessment of the fluid deficit which may be confirmed by the degree of elevation of the packed cell volume and the concentration and electrolyte content of the urine. It must be emphasised that haematocrit readings are only reliable in the early acute phase of obstruction and in the absence of haemorrhage. The volume lost should be replaced by giving isotonic saline with the addition of 1 g (13 mEq) of potassium chloride to each litre. Hypertonic sodium chloride should be given if the serum sodium level is low and plasma expanders used if circulatory failure has developed. Half the total deficit should be given during 3 to 4 hours and the rate of infusion of the remainder determined by the response obtained. The rate of infusion in the elderly and in those with cardiopulmonary insufficiency should be controlled by observing changes in central venous pressure.

When obstruction has developed slowly due to granulomatous disease of the intestine the picture is often different. Electrolytes pass more easily into the lumen of the gut if it is inflamed and diarrhoea may precede obstruction in conditions like Crohn's disease. Sodium, potassium and magnesium will thus be lost early as well as water. The fall in potassium and magnesium levels may lead to paralysis of the intestine with further aggravation of the initial problems. Hypoalbuminaemia may also have developed as a result of the primary pathology and will contribute to further electrolyte losses into oedema fluid.

Fistulae

The metabolic consequences of intestinal fistulae depend upon the site of the fistulae. Fluid and electrolyte depletion occurs rapidly in duodenal fistulae and slowly, if at all, with ileal lesions.

The principles of management of all intestinal fistulae are first the collection and measurement of losses so that adequate replacement can be prescribed. A search must then be undertaken for any associated intraabdominal abscesses which should be drained. The nutritional state must be maintained by parenteral feeding and when a state of metabolic balance has been reached the exact site of the fistula and the presence or absence of distal obstruction can be determined radiologically. If there is no obstruction beyond the fistula, much can be gained by waiting and over half of such fistulae in the small bowel will close spontaneously (Chapman, 1964). The importance of nutrition in the management is emphasised by the high mortality when significant malnutrition was present (Edmonds et al, 1960).

Early operation has been advocated for high small bowel fistulae but recurrence rates are high if early closure is attempted. Definitive operation for fistulae must include a full dissection mobilisation and resection of the affected segment with end-to-end anastomosis. Patience is necessary in the management of all intestinal fistulae to achieve metabolic balance and healthy granulations in the wound before careful and deliberate surgery is undertaken.

Oesophagogastric Fistula

This is a well recognised complication of surgery of the lower oesophagus or gastric fundus. The volumes of fluid coming from the fistula can be great and will contain a high concentration of H^+. All oral feeding should cease when the fistula opens and full parenteral feeding commenced to reduce the amount of gastric secretion. A proportion will close spontaneously provided nutritional and electrolyte balance is maintained.

Duodenal Fistula

The commonest cause of this fistula was rupture of the duodenal stump following polya gastrectomy. The decline in popularity of gastrectomy has led to a reduction in numbers of duodenal fistulae. The mortality from this complication was high mainly due to the large volumes (2–3 litres) of fluid lost daily, which can rapidly prove fatal if uncorrected. The average daily composition of duodenal secretions are shown in Table 30.

Gastrojejunocolic Fistula

This complication of recurrent ulceration after partial gastrectomy is now uncommon. The condition also develops when carcinoma of the stomach invades the colon. Diarrhoea and weight loss can be the main symptoms in many and pain may be absent. Some patients may vomit foul material. The infestation of the upper small intestine with faecal organisms leads to inflammation of the jejunal mucosa and the breakdown of fats to abnormal fatty acids. Diarrhoea is due to a combination of causes. The urinary Indican level is often raised indicating abnormal bacterial colonisation of the small intestine. Steatorrhoea, creatorrhoea and Vitamin K lack occur. Treatment initially with antibiotics will reduce the diarrhoea and improve intestinal absorption. Infusions of albumin and parenteral feeding will be required preparatory to surgical correction of the fistula (French and Crane, 1963).

Biliary Fistula

Partial biliary fistulae are common for a few days after operations on the common bile duct but total fistulae are relatively uncommon. The daily losses of bile are about 500 to 700 ml from a total fistula. Bile is alkaline with a bicarbonate concentration of 40 mEq/litre. The principal losses however are sodium (140 mEq/L) and chloride (90 mEq/L) and these may be overlooked. The daily losses must be replaced either intravenously or by giving sodium chloride capsules orally. When total biliary fistulae persist the reduced absorption of Vitamin K and diminished prothrombin formation must not be overlooked. The problem of ascending infection in prolonged fistulae must also be remembered.

Pancreatic Fistulae

Excoriation and digestion of the wound occur early in pancreatic fistulae due to the digestive enzymes in the secretions. Silicone barrier creams, milk powder with sump drainage of the fistula or, on the other hand, nursing the patient in the prone position are all useful means of controlling skin digestion. The metabolic problems of a pancreatic fistula are due mainly to the hypertonic nature of pancreatic secretions. The pancreatic cells actively secrete bicarbonate and sodium and the fluid lost may contain up to 180 mEq/litre of bicarbonate and 170 mEq/ litre of sodium (Moore, 1962). Replacement with isotonic saline will lead to overloading with water and sodium depletion. The serum pH falls due to the loss of base. Replacement with sodium bicarbonate and lactate is required and hypertonic saline may be necessary.

Intestinal Fistulae

In high fistulae fluid and electrolyte losses overshadow any nutritional problems and were considered formerly as an indication for early surgery. Any attempt to feed orally patients with jejunal fistulae leads to further fluid losses even though some nutrients may be absorbed above the fistula. The introduction of a feeding jejunostomy beyond the fistula can be most valuable. This enables the nutritional requirements and the drainage from the fistula to be passed on to absorptive surfaces of the distal bowel.

The fluid and electrolyte losses from intestinal fistula are related to the composition of normal intestinal contents (Table 30). Allowance should always be made for sodium losses of at least 120 mEq per litre; Potassium losses will be about 15 mEq per litre and will be higher if granulomatous disease is present in the small intestine. Acid base imbalance will only occur in high jejunal fistulae when the serum pH and standard bicarbonate will fall gradually if replacement is inadequate.

Intestinal fistulae may also be internal in association with granulomatous diseases of the bowel. Jejunocolic or ileojejunal fistulae will produce bacterial contamination of the absorptive area of the small intestine and metabolic competition, steatorrhoea and weight loss will then ensue. The presence of large numbers of organisms in the jejunum can be detected by measuring the amount of indocyanic acid (Indican) present in the urine. This substance is produced by the metabolism of tryptophan in the gut by the organisms. Situations such as internal fistulae or blind loops require antibiotic control as a prelude to surgical correction.

Ileostomy

This is a surgical fistula which normally produces no problems but occasionally excessive losses occur in the first few days after the ileostomy is made. The electrolyte concentration of ileal fluid is about 110 mEq sodium and 5 to 10 mEq of potassium per litre. The potassium losses in the early stages may be higher due to inflammation of the ileum associated with ulcerative colitis (Brooke and Slaney, 1967).

High daily outputs of fluid in excess of one litre can soon lead to hyponatraemia and hypovolaemia. A high output usually suggests the presence of subacute obstruction or the development of intraperitoneal sepsis.

REFERENCES

Howe, C. T. and Le Quesne, L. P. (1964). Pyloric stenosis. The metabolic effect. *Brit. J. Surg.* **51**, 923.

Shields, R. (1964). Surgical aspects of the absorption of water and electrolytes by the intestine. Monographs in surgical science. Vol. 1 Baltimore. The Williams & Williams Co. 119–171.

Chapman, R., Foran, R. and Dunply, J. E. (1964). Management of intestinal fistulae. *Amer. J. Surg.* **108**, 157.

Edmunds, L. H., Williams, G. M. and Welds, C. E. (1960). External fistulae arising from the gastrointestinal tract. *Ann. Surg.* **152**, 445.

French, J. M. and Crane, C. W. (1963). Undernutrition, malnutrition and malabsorption after gastrectomy in partial gastrectomy. Complications and metabolic consequences. Stammers, F. A. R. and Williams, J. A. (Editors). London, Butterworths.

Moore, F. D. (1962). Regulation of the serum sodium concentrations. *Amer. J. Surg.* **103**, 302.

Brooke, B. N. and Slaney, G. (1967). Metabolic Derangements in gastro-intestinal surgery. American lecture series. Charles C. Thomas, Springfield, Ill.

Booth, C. C., MacIntyre, I. and Nollen, D. C. (1964). Nutritional problems associated with extensive lesions of the distal small intestine in man. *Quart. J. Med.* **33**, 401.

Johnston, I. D. A. (1970). The management of side effects of surgery for peptic ulceration. *Brit. J. Surg.* **57**, 787.

12: Intestinal Malabsorption

Many conditions can cause malabsorption of nutrients (Table 31). Conditions which are of surgical interest will be discussed. Weight loss and diarrhoea are the usual indications that malabsorption is present and the presence of more than 5 g of fat in the stool each day is further evidence of the problem.

Table 31

Some Causes of Intestinal Malabsorption

A. *Surgical*
1. Resection of small bowel
2. Gastric surgery
3. Enterocutaneous fistulae

B. *Bacterial Contamination*
1. Blind loops
2. Enterocolic fistulae
3. Jejunal diverticulosis
4. Strictures

C. *Mucosal Lesions*
1. Crohn's disease
2. Coeliac disease and idiopathic steatorrhoea
3. Infiltrative lesions (amyloid, reticuloses, etc.)

D. *Vascular Lesions*
1. Superior mesenteric artery occlusion.

1. Massive Resection

The patient who has had a massive resection of the small intestine because of thromboembolic, neoplastic or granulomatous disease presents a considerable nutritional and metabolic problem. The problem consists of providing the necessary fluid requirements and giving every opportunity for absorption of nutrients when the absorptive surfaces are reduced and transit time increased.

Resection of the distal intestine is performed more often than proximal resection. With resection of terminal ileum alone the absorption of B_{12} is reduced. When the excision is more extensive steatorrhoea and loss of protein will be present in addition to malabsorption of B_{12}.

With massive ileal resection malabsorption of all nutrients can be detected. Resection of the proximal intestine is better tolerated than removal of the distal bowel and unless resection is massive the distal intestine takes over the functions of the resected proximal intestine. It is possible to maintain patients with up to 80% resection of the small intestine in reasonably good condition. There have been a number of reports of patients surviving for variable periods with as little as 6 to 8 in of jejunum.

Immediately after massive resection diarrhoea is a serious problem, fluid and electrolyte depletion occurs and hypokalaemia with muscle weakness has been observed (Booth et al, 1964). The initial diarrhoea subsides and provided there is an adequate length of colon, electrolyte problems are resolved and give way to nutritional deficiencies. Compensatory hypertrophy does occur and is maximal after 6 months. Patients with no more than 2 feet of jejunum may pass a single formed stool per day. When steatorrhoea is present the absorption of calcium will be reduced and hypocalcaemia, tetany and magnesium depletion may all develop after massive resection. The malabsorption of protein is never so extensive as that for fat but hypoproteinaemia may develop gradually.

Nutritional Care

Patients with resection require considerable nutritional support. Initially parenteral nutrition is necessary as it is easier to maintain body weight by parenteral means rather than restore weight that has been lost. Later albumin and blood infusions may be needed from time to time depending on the extent of the resection. Injections of B_{12} and iron are also essential to maintain normal haemopoiesis. The capabilities of the residual intestine must be assessed regularly.

The low bulk liquid diet designed for the American space programme has proved useful in patients with intestinal insufficiency (Thompson et al, 1969). This liquid or chemical diet consisting of L amino acids, glucose, minerals and medium chain triglycerides (Winitz et al, 1965) can maintain nutrition in normal subjects for long periods of time. These nutrients produce minimal stimulation of the pancreas and biliary system and can be absorbed rapidly. The unpalatable nature of most chemical diets is a distinct disadvantage.

The concentration of solute in liquid feeds requires frequent adjustment according to the tolerance of the intestine to changes in osmolality. The administration of codeine phosphate will enable more concentrated solutions to be given.

Massive resection of the small intestine has been followed by greatly increased secretion of gastric acid (Osborne et al, 1967) due to the loss of normal inhibitory mechanisms in the resected bowel. It has been suggested that perhaps the vagi should be divided at the time of bowel resection to control this oversecretion of acid but there is little support for this procedure from current clinical experience.

Some patients with moderate resections of intestine who have intractable diarrhoea may be improved by a subsequent reversal of a short segment 10–12 cm of lower small intestine. This procedure, which is not without its hazards, will reduce transit time and improve intestinal absorption and nutrition (Craft & Venables, 1968).

2. Protein losing Enteropathy

Hypoproteinaemia and oedema develop occasionally due to the abnormal loss of protein into the gut. Apart from ulcerative colitis and Crohn's disease, carcinoma of the stomach, idiopathic steatorrhoea and giant hypertrophy of gastric folds are other conditions which cause abnormal losses of protein into the bowel. The liver is incapable of synthesising enough albumin to make up for the losses even though the protein lost is reabsorbed as amino acids. Several methods of detecting the abnormality are available. The intravenous injection of ^{51}Cr albumin is used. After passage into the bowel the ^{51}Cr is broken off from the albumin but is not reabsorbed and can be measured.

3. Crohn's Disease

Chronic granulomatous conditions of the bowel or Crohn's disease may affect large sections of the small intestine and malabsorption in this condition depends upon the extent of the disease as well as complicating factors such as previous resections, strictures or fistulae. The faecal losses of nitrogen under these conditions may be as great as 10 g of nitrogen daily and the alimentary canal can be a major protein losing area (Fig. 40). Malabsorption for fat and B_{12} is also usually present in extensive Crohn's disease. Some patients with advanced Crohn's disease find it difficult to maintain an adequate nutritional state.

4. Ulcerative Colitis

The profuse watery diarrhoea in colitis may lead at first to electrolyte disorders rather than nutritional deficiencies and as much as 70 to 80 mEq of potassium may be lost daily during an exacerbation. Much of this loss is due to leakage of potassium from damaged mucosal cells in the colon. Sodium losses can also be high and amount to more than 200 mEq per day. Malabsorption is not usually associated with ulcerative colitis unless complications such as amyloid disease are present. However, considerable protein losses amounting to 60–70 g (10 g nitrogen) daily may occur from the ulcerated area of the colon. The plasma protein levels fall gradually in the face of prolonged alimentary losses of protein. Many patients with colitis have a poor intake of food during exacerbations and thus lose weight.

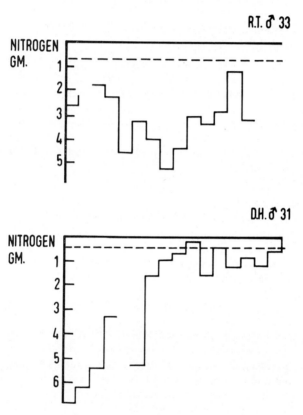

FIG. 40. Faecal Nitrogen losses in Crohn's disease during intravenous feeding alone.

5. Bacterial Competition

Nutritional disorders develop in patients with a variety of lesions in the small intestine which allow the development of an abnormal bacterial flora in stagnant segments. Reference has been made to fistulae. Other conditions include enteroanastomoses, blind loops and a partially obstructed afferent duodenal loop after polya gastrectomy. The level of indican in the urine is usually high.

The improvement in intestinal absorption which follows treatment with antibiotics in patients with blind loops or strictures emphasises the role of bacteria. The mechanism of bacterial induced malabsorption may be related to the toxic action of the bacterial breakdown products from bile salts acting on the intestinal mucosa (Dawson and Isselbackher, 1960).

Miscellaneous Causes of Watery Diarrhoea

1. Staphylococcal Diarrhoea

This is a serious complication of surgery in which rapid large losses of fluid occur into the bowel causing hypovolaemia and collapse. The diarrhoea is blood stained and organisms can be identified by gram staining and microscopy. The immediate requirement is the intravenous infusion of isotonic saline and large amounts must be given quickly to keep pace with the massive transfer of sodium into the lumen of the bowel. A potassium deficit will soon follow in severe cases and colloid is also required.

2. Villous Adenoma

Large villous adenomas of the lower colon can produce a profound metabolic disorder due to diarrhoea and electrolyte loss (Fig. 41). Patients may be admitted in a semicomatose state due to dehydration, hyponatraemia and hypokalaemia with an associated increase in the blood urea. Base is lost mainly and the serum pH and standard bicarbonate levels are low denoting a metabolic acidosis. These patients have often been passing several watery stools daily for many months. The volume of the stools increases gradually and 2 to 3 litres of fluid may be lost in 24 hours. Duthie and Atwell (1963) showed that the nett movement of sodium and water was reversed and the secretion of potassium increased in villous papillomas. The rectal fluid in this condition may contain as much as 150 mEq per litre of sodium and 80 mEq per litre potassium. Fluid and electrolyte balance must be restored before any operation to remove the tumour is undertaken.

3. Endocrine Causes of Diarrhoea

Diarrhoea may be the presenting feature of the rare α cell tumours of the pancreas. Two separate syndromes have been described. Some patients with gastric hypersecretion, recurrent peptic ulceration and α cell tumours have severe diarrhoea and steatorrhoea. Inactivation of lipase by excessive acid secretion is suggested as a cause of the diarrhoea. A second syndrome is now recognised in which profuse watery diarrhoea occurs in the presence of gastric achlorhydria and no peptic ulceration. These patients develop a severe potassium and

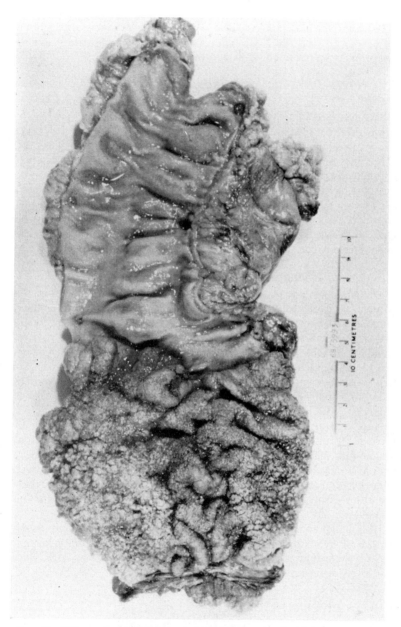

F<small>IG</small>. 41. Villous adenoma of rectum which was associated with hypokalaemia,
hyponatraemia and a raised blood urea.

sodium deficiency. The pancreatic tumour contains a hormone with properties of secretin (Zollinger, 1969).

Patients with carcinoid tumours and hepatic metastases also often have severe diarrhoea and hypokalaemia. This symptom responds occasionally to treatment with serotonin antagonists.

4. Uretero-Intestinal Anastomosis

Odel and Ferris (1951) found that patients with ureterosigmoidostomy often developed a hyperchloraemic acidosis. Healthy kidneys are able to compensate for the colonic reabsorption of urinary sodium and chloride but, if the kidney becomes damaged as a result of ascending infection, it becomes unable to secrete urine with a low pH. Urinary potassium is not reabsorbed from the colon and, when large quantities of urine are passing through the colon, hypokalaemia develops. Treatment consists of the intravenous infusion of sodium bicarbonate or citrate with concurrent administration of potassium. Sufficient fluid must be given to induce a diuresis, keeping the acid base and electrolyte balance under surveillance.

5. General Management

The management of patients with abnormal fluid losses from the alimentary canal must be based on the measurement of the daily volumes lost and its concentration of sodium, potassium, bicarbonate and chloride. Measurement of the blood urea and the plasma pH and standard bicarbonate will also assist in planning intravenous replacement. The nutritional state must be maintained by the appropriate adjuvant use of intravenous nutrients or elemental diets when required, but nutritional needs must take second place to fluid and electrolyte balance.

Any consideration of alimentary losses either from diarrhoea or through fistulae must take into account the alimentary control of magnesium balance. Magnesium is a divalent intracellular cation sharing some of the properties of calcium and potassium. The normal concentration in plasma is 1·5 to 2·0 mEq/litre. About 60% of the daily excretion of magnesium is in the faeces and the body requires about 200 mg per day in the diet (Chapter 2).

Hypomagnesaemia is difficult to detect clinically as it is often associated with hypokalaemia. Central nervous system irritability, altered E.C.G. recordings and poor protein synthesis are all associated with low levels of serum magnesium.

Effects of Gastric Surgery

Gastric operations are followed in a number of patients by early and late complications which are of metabolic significance. The early side effects of surgery consist of a series of symptoms related to eating.

The late side effects are nutritional and are due mainly to a diminished intake of food.

Early Side Effects

Dumping

The dumping symptom complex of faintness, sweating, trembling and tachycardia during and after meals is noticed almost immediately after surgery. Nausea, the feeling of fullness and, on occasions, diarrhoea soon after a meal are other components of dumping. The symptoms in one form or another afflict between 5 and 15% of patients following even vagotomy and drainage operations (Cox, 1968). The symptoms are less severe after vagotomy compared to gastrectomy but nevertheless 1% of patients remain handicapped by dumping as long as 20 years after vagotomy (Wheldon et al, 1969).

Dumping is usually associated with a diminished plasma volume. Large amounts of glucose in the jejunum induce osmotic movement of fluid into the lumen. It was thought that there is a block in utilisation of glucose during dumping and that this hindered the absorption of further glucose.

Tolbutamide 250–500 mg given half an hour before meals has been used to stimulate insulin release and enhance glucose transport into the cell. This treatment is effective in some patients. A slow insulin release and failure of glucose utilisation is however only part of the problem. Symptoms can occur and the blood volume can fall even when there is a brisk rise in plasma insulin after stimulation (Fig. 42). Other factors, such as the release of serotonin from the jejunum and the neurogenic response to distension, have been implicated as causing dumping (Johnston, 1970).

Bilious Vomiting

Bilious vomiting is induced when bile regurgitates into stomachs sensitive to the presence of bile. This symptom like dumping becomes less severe as time passes. Surgical conversion procedures which divert bile from the stomach are valuable in over 90% of patients with bilious vomiting who remain seriously handicapped by the symptoms. Drugs like metochlopramide which increase the rate of gastric emptying may be effective in controlling bilious vomiting.

Diarrhoea

Diarrhoea is uncommon after gastrectomy but three types occur following vagotomy. Transitory diarrhoea appears in the first few weeks after surgery and clears up spontaneously in most patients. Episodic diarrhoea in which several loose stools are passed may occur at irregular intervals. The attacks are of short duration, sudden in onset and incontinence may be present.

Continuous diarrhoea or a constant increase in frequency of bowel action may be severe enough to be really incapacitating.

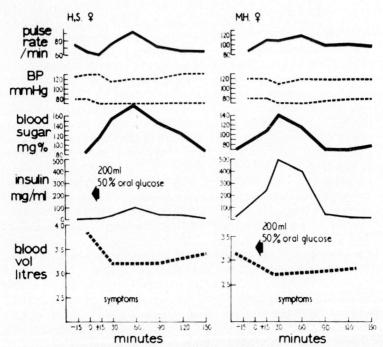

.—Dumping after vagotomy and pyloroplasty indicating that symptoms and cardiovascular changes can occur with a marked increase in plasma-insulin levels.

FIG. 42. Plasma Insulin in dumping syndrome.

Continuous diarrhoea or increased frequency is associated with weight loss and probably impaired fat absorption. Episodic diarrhoea is not related to loss of weight. A few patients with severe and crippling diarrhoea may have their intestinal transit time reduced by the reversal of a short segment of ileum. There is no specific remedy for post vagotomy diarrhoea but simple measures such as codeine phosphate or diphenoxylate (Lomotil) are sometimes helpful.

Late Side Effects

Weight Loss

Some of the nutritional consequences of gastric surgery develop insidiously over a number of years. Many of the late metabolic problems can be prevented and they should be recognised in patients who have had gastric surgery in the past.

Many patients lose weight after gastrectomy or vagotomy and drainage procedures. The extent of the weight loss is related to the presence or absence of post-cibal symptoms and the ability to eat full meals.

Anaemia

Iron deficiency anaemia develops within the first 5 years of gastric surgery in a significant number of patients, particularly women. Anaemia is not related to weight changes or post-cibal symptoms. The serum B_{12} level falls gradually after gastric surgery and the absorption of B_{12} is reduced, and can be restored to normal by the addition of intrinsic factor.

Bone Disease

Metabolic bone disease is a well recognised problem after gastrectomy and 2-4% of patients have evidence of osteomalacia after 5 or more years. The serum calcium is low and the alkaline phosphatase is raised in many. It is not certain whether these biochemical changes indicate impending osteomalacia. Metabolic bone disease has not been recorded so far after vagotomy and drainage operations although the biochemical changes can be detected after 15 years in between 4 and 6% of patients.

Severe hypoproteinaemia with nutritional oedema and Vitamin B deficiency has been recorded after gastrectomy but severe nutritional disorders have not been observed following vagotomy.

Regular dietetic advice with supplemental iron and on occasions Vitamin D can prevent nutritional inadequacy after gastric surgery.

Pancreatitis

Pancreatitis is a serious disorder which produces profound metabolic disturbances. The principal problem is a rapid and severe loss of circulating blood volume due to the loss of plasma into the pancreas and neighbouring tissues and as much as 30% of the blood volume may be lost in a few hours (Moore, 1959). The packed cell volume may be raised if plasma is mainly lost. The management of hypovolaemic shock has been discussed in Chapter VI and the restoration of blood volume and elevation of the blood pressure is of prime importance.

Immediate Problems

Acute inflammation in the retroperitoneal space can cause a secondary paralytic ileus and further quantities of fluid may be isolated in segments of paralysed small intestine. Replacement therapy must consist therefore of a combination of blood plasma or plasma substitute and isotonic saline. The rate of infusion should be judged among other things by the volume of urine produced. Potassium is not usually required initially. The serum amylase levels reach a peak within the first 24 hours and fall thereafter. Serum amylase levels also rise but much more slowly in other upper abdominal inflammatory conditions. Normal levels of serum amylase may be present with acute pancreatitis and high levels may be associated with other acute abdominal conditions such as perforated peptic ulcer.

The level of serum calcium falls in 70% of patients with pancreatitis within the first few days. Soaps formed in areas of tissue destruction and fat necrosis take up a lot of calcium and the serum calcium may fall and tetany develop. Low serum calcium levels carry a poor prognosis. The serum calcium level should be measured regularly in pancreatitis and calcium gluconate given when required.

Magnesium can also be incoporated into soaps and the level in blood may be reduced.

Pancreatitis may develop after operations in the stomach, duodenum or biliary system. If is often not recognised in the immediate post-operative period, when it is difficult to distinguish from paralytic ileus. Postoperative pancreatitis carries a high mortality rate (Foster and Ziffren, 1962).

Chronic Problems

Chronic relapsing pancreatitis is associated with metabolic disturbances. Half the patients will develop glucose intolerance and about 40% will develop steatorrhoea with associated malabsorption problems and hypocalcaemia. The management of pancreatic failure due either to pancreatitis or resection of the pancreas requires the addition of pancreatic enzymes to the diet to prevent an intestinal malabsorption developing. It is very difficult to abolish steatorrhoea completely, but daily intake of 12 g pancreatin by mouth will reduce the faecal nitrogen and fat by about 50%.

A few patients have survived for many years after total pancreatectomy (Whitfield et al, 1965). The diabetic state which follows pancreatic resection is easy to control and the vascular and neurological complications of diabetes do not occur in these patients.

REFERENCES

Thompson, W. R., Stevens, R. V., Randell, H. T. and Bowen, J. R. (1969). The space diet in the management of a patient with extreme short bowel syndrome. *Amer. J. Surg.* **117,** 449.

Winitz, M., Fraff, J., Gallagher, N., Harkin, A. and Seedman, D. (1965). Chemical diets as nutrition for man in space. *Nature* **205,** 741.

Osborne, M. P., Sizer, T., Frederick, P. L. and Zamcheck, M. (1967). Massive bowel resection and gastric hypersecretion. *Amer. J. Surg.* **114**, 393.

Craft, I. L. and Venables, C. W. (1968). Reversed jejunal segment for intestinal hurry. *Ann. Surg.* **167**, 282.

Dawson, A. M. and Isselbacher, K. J. (1960). Studies on lipid metabolism in the small intestine with observations on the role of bile salts. *J. Clin. Invest.* **39**, 730.

Duthie, H. L. and Atwell, J. D. (1963). The absorption of water, sodium and potassium in the large intestine with reference to villous adenoma. *Gut* **4**, 373.

Zollinger, R. M., Tompkins, R. K., Amerson, R. J., Endahl, G. T., Kraft, A. T. and Moore, F. T. (1968). Secretin like substances in islet cell tumours of the pancreas. *Ann. Surg.* **168**, 502.

Shields, R. (1964). Surgical aspects of the absorption of water and electrolytes by the intestine. *Monographs in the Surgical Sciences.* **1**, 119.

William, J. A. and Cox, A. (1969). After Vagotomy. Butterworths.

Wheldon, E. J., Venables, C. W. and Johnston, I. D. A. (1970). Late metabolic consequences of vagotomy and gastroenterostomy. *Lancet* **1**, 437.

Moore, F. D. (1959). Metabolic care of the surgical patient. Philadelphia. W. B. Saunders Co.

Whitfield, A. G. W., Crane, C. N., French, J. M. and Bayley, T. J. Life without a pancreas. *Lancet* **1**, 675.

13: Management of Nutritional Problems

Intravenous Feeding

The nutrition of surgical patients can often be overlooked due to the pressing demands of other more urgent needs. Many surgical patients can benefit from the intravenous administration of nutrients while others whose alimentary canal cannot be used for variable periods of time require intravenous feeding if they are to survive. The effect of giving parenteral nutrients in the few days after uncomplicated surgery in well nourished patients has been considered (Chapter III). The concept of intravenous nutrition is not a new one. Hodder, writing in the Lancet in 1873, described the intravenous infusion of milk as a source of nourishment in patients with cholera. These early attempts of parenteral feeding were unsuccessful and glucose solutions became the mainstay of parenteral nutrition for many years but one litre of 5% glucose can only provide 200 calories. Amino acids have been available for intravenous use since 1937 and are available as whole protein hydrolysates or mixtures of synthetic amino acids. It is now possible to provide all the daily requirements of fat protein and carbohydrate by the intravenous route and maintain the nutritional state of patients for quite long periods. The management of effective parenteral feeding, however, requires considerable attention to detail. The salient features of the preparations available will be described and the advantages as well as the complications in various clinical situations outlined.

Amino Acids

Protein is necessary in any feeding programme and amino acids are thus essential in parenteral feeding to maintain the balance of nitrogen and form new protein.

Henriques and Anderson (1913) carried out the first successful intravenous feeding programme using amino acids. Their mixture consisted of a digest of goat muscle by intestinal enzymes, glucose and a mixture of sodium, potassium and magnesium salts was added to the extract. This solution was then infused intravenously at a steady rate as the only source of nourishment and the animals were found to

212

remain in positive nitrogen balance during the study. The essential amino acids were subsequently identified, but nothing more was done about their combination for parenteral use until 1939, when Elman, in St. Louis, observed that the infusion of 5% amino acid mixture and 5% glucose in dogs following injury produced greater plasma protein regeneration than when 10% glucose was used alone. The amino acid solution used was a sulphuric acid hydrolysate of casein to which Tryptophan and Cystine were added.

Intravenous amino acids are not incorporated into body protein unless there is a simultaneous supply of exogenous calories, some of which must be available from carbohydrate sources (Munro, 1963). The proportion of infused amino acids utilised is related to the number of calories available, but more information is required on calorie Nitrogen ratios under varying conditions.

Two types of amino acid solutions have been developed for clinical use. The enzymatic hydrolysis of the whole protein casein produces a mixture of essential amino acids and peptides of varying molecular size, depending on the extent of the hydrolysis. Large molecular peptides are removed by dialysis. The remaining solution has no antigenic properties and can maintain nitrogen equilibrium in both man and animals. Casein hydrolysates contain about 66% of free amino acids and 33% peptides and the 3·3% solution which is used widely has about 4·5 g of nitrogen per litre.

Recently mixtures of pure crystalline amino acids have been prepared for intravenous use. One such mixture contains 10 amino acids, eight of which are essential. The total nitrogen and amino nitrogen concentration of these synthetic mixtures are higher than in the 3·3% casein hydrolysate solution. The pH is higher and is about 7·0. This may be an advantage in reducing the amount of vein irritation. The composition of preparations available and daily minimal requirements of amino acids are shown in Table 32. The body may be able to utilise all the nitrogen in any amino acid mixture but there is no doubt the α amino nitrogen is the most readily available source and accurate studies should take account of both amino and total nitrogen.

The value of infused amino acids depends on various factors. Some amino acids are excreted rapidly; some are metabolised to produce energy and others are converted to body protein. The essential amino acids must be given in a ratio similar to that in whole protein for the most efficient utilisation to occur. The necessity for the simultaneous infusion of calories has led to the preparation of mixtures containing fructose, sorbitol, and alcohol, along with the amino acids.

With the exception of D methionine and D phenylalanine the body can only utilise the laevo rotatory or L form of any amino acid.

The hydrolysis of a whole protein to produce a solution of amino acids for intravenous use leads to a number of problems. Alkali hydrolysis degrades some amino acids and the result is a mixture of the D and L forms. When enzymes are used there is a large residue of peptides in the solutions and these may account for some of the side effects such as nausea or pyrexia which occasionally follow infusion of casein hydrolysates.

Table 32.
Requirements of Essential Amino Acids and Composition of some Amino Acid Solutions at Present Available

	Minimal Daily requirements of essential amino acids in adult human (gm)	Synthetic D and L amino acid (Trophysan) 10% (gm/L)	Composition of average casein hydrolysate (Aminosol) 10% (gm/L)	Synthetic L amino acid (Vamin) 7% (gm/L)
Threonine	0·50	1·4	3·9	3·0
Valine	0·80	1·9	6·0	4·3
Methione	1·10	2·2	3·1	1·9
Isoleucine	0·70	1·4	5·0	3·9
Leucine	1·10	2·2	9·8	5·3
Phenylalanine	1·10	1·9	5·2	5·5
Tryptophan	0·25	0·8	1·0	1·0
Lysine	0·80	3·3	7·2	3·9
Histidine			2·1	2·4
Arginine		1·0	4·1	3·3
Glycine		2·5	1·9	2·1
a-amino-N		6·5	7·5	7·8
Total N		6·7	12·7	9·4

Mixtures of synthetic D and L amino acids (Trophysan) have been available for some time and glycine is added frequently as a source of non-essential amino acid. Studies in the postoperative period show that the preparation Trophysan is not as effective in maintaining the balance of nitrogen as Casein hydrolysates or mixtures of synthetic L amino acids. Mixtures of synthetic L amino acids would appear to be ideal and they have recently become available. Preliminary studies indicate their superiority over synthetic D and L mixtures. However, there is little difference between the new synthetic mixtures and casein hydrolysates which will probably remain popular for some time (Tweedle and Johnston, 1971). Synthetic L amino acids should be free from side effects and situations which demand high quality control such as the management of neonatal problems will benefit from the use of synthetic mixtures.

Blood and Plasma

Blood or plasma is of no immediate value from a nutritional point of view. Plasma proteins are deficient in tryptophan and isoleucine and it takes many weeks for significant amounts of amino acids derived from infused plasma proteins to be reincorporated into body protein. Blood, albumin or plasma infusions must be given only to restore plasma levels of protein quickly if the levels are very low or continued protein losses are anticipated.

Fat

By far the most important advance in parenteral nutrition has been the development of safe and stable fat solutions (Edgren and Wretlind, 1963).

In normal nutrition, fat releases 9·3 calories for each gram utilised, and normally about 30% of the total calorie requirements comes from fat. The intravenous administration of suitable fat emulsions has many attractions. Large numbers of calories can be given in small volumes of fluid, there are no harmful byproducts left after metabolism and osmotic effects are negligible as fat is not a true solution even in high concentrations. Stability of the solutions and side effects after infusion have, however, been major problems in the development of a suitable preparation for routine use.

Short chain triglycerides were found to be very toxic and preparations of either Soya bean or cottonseed oil have been found to be the most satisfactory.

The problem of producing a stable fat emulsion was first tackled by Japanese workers about 1920 and they had some success using lecithin as an emulsifying agent in Soya bean oil. The introduction of Soya bean phosphatide as an emulsifying agent led to the preparation of solutions both of cottonseed and Soya bean oil suitable for clinical use, but is was not until 1957 that Wretlind and his colleagues prepared a fat emulsion that was completely safe for clinical use. A particle size of 1 micron was achieved initially by these methods. The preparations available today have a particle size of 0·5 μ and are consequently more stable.

Halberg and his colleagues (1966), found that cottonseed oil emulsions were much more toxic, both in animals and man, than Soya bean oil preparations. This toxicity was considered to be due to the presence of an impurity (Gossypol) in the cottonseed emulsions and these preparations were withdrawn from clinical use. Most experience with intravenous fat has been obtained using Soya bean oil emulsions and this preparation can be given safely for prolonged periods to ill patients. Cottonseed oil emulsions have been reintroduced following removal of the toxic element but the full clinical evaluation of this preparation must await further study. Soya bean oil contains more linolenic acid and less saturated fatty acids than cottonseed oil and glucose or glycerol is added to the water phase of the emulsion to make the solution isotonic with plasma. The formulae for the two main types of fat emulsion available today are shown in Table 33.

Fat injected intravenously is metabolised rapidly by the body and 70% of the carbon of infused fat appears as carbon dioxide in the lungs within 4 hours. The rate of removal of infused fat from the bloodstream is similar to the rate of removal of chylomicrons from orally administered fat (Lawson, 1965).

Table 33.

Composition of Fat Emulsions

	Lipiphysan	Intralipid (20%)
Soyabean oil		200 G
Cottonseed oil	150 G	
Soyabean phosphatides	15 G	
Sorbitol	50 G	
Egg yolk phosphatides		12 G
Glycerol		25 G
Distilled water	1000 ml	1000 ml

Fat emulsions have no antigenic properties and acute toxicity is very rare. When fat infusions of 3–4 g per kg are given at a time, backache, headache, rigors and pyrexia have been reported occasionally during administration. Calories from intravenous fat preparations can replace oral supplements in the maintenance of body weight. Lawson (1965) gave 3 g per kg per day for periods of 18 to 36 days and found no biochemical of any liver dysfunction and liver biopsies taken after 30 and 36 days of infusions showed no abnormality of liver cell structure. Very prolonged infusions have been reported to cause haemolytic anaemia, thrombocytopenia and prolonged coagulation time in some patients. The presence of fat particles in plasma reduces capillary circulation. The effect on the microcirculation of the kidney in man is not known but no changes have been observed in glomerular filtration rate during prolonged infusions of fat. Fat emulsions are not irritant to veins and indeed may be used in combination with more irritant fluids. Heparin is added sometimes to parenteral fat solutions on the assumption that it will accelerate lipase activity and enhance fat clearance from the plasma.

Alcohol

Alcohol is an important calorie source in parenteral dietetics and has an energy value greater than that of carbohydrate. One gram of alcohol provides 7·1 calories and a litre of 5% solution about 350 calories. Ethyl alcohol (Ethanol) is used in parenteral feeding and can be infused at a rate of 10 g (70 calories) per hour in a 3 or 5% solution without at the same time inducing undue side effects. Some patients will experience a slight euphoria which may be beneficial. Others will experience drowsiness and disorientation. Patients differ greatly in their tolerance to intravenous alcohol. Females have a lower limit of tolerance and very high blood levels occur rapidly if liver function is abnormal. Fat may accumulate in the liver and ultra structural cellular changes have been reported following ethanol infusions.

Amino acids have been shown to increase the rate of elimination of alcohol from the blood. Carbohydrate is also required for the complete oxidation of infused alcohol to acetaldehyde which is oxidised finally through the tricarboxylic acid cycle to give CO_2 and water.

Carbohydrate

Glucose remains an important calorie source in any parenteral feeding programme. There is a limit, however, to the number of calories which can be provided by glucose in any programme of intravenous feeding. One litre of 5% glucose will only provide 200 calories. The blood concentration of glucose should not exceed the renal threshold if water, electrolyte and calorie loss through diuresis is to be avoided. Glucose in a concentration of 5% has a pH of about 4·0 and this may be a potent cause of thrombophlebitis. Higher concentrations of carbohydrate solutions usually cause severe vein irritation and thrombosis and it is probably the osmolality of solutions which are the major factors in causing phlebitis.

Fructose is an attractive alternative source of carbohydrate. It also escapes in the urine at high concentrations and the urinary losses of glucose and fructose are similar. Fructose is metabolised much more rapidly by the body than glucose. Fructose metabolism takes place mainly in the liver in contrast to the peripheral utilisation of glucose and is largely independent of insulin and unaffected by adenocorticosteroids.

In postoperative patients 40% of an infusion of fructose is utilised in the liver, while 12% goes to form muscle glycogen. Glucose on the other hand is used mainly in the peripheral tissues when 30% is converted to muscle glycogen and only 15% utilised in the liver. Some fructose is converted to glucose during metabolism and there is a rise in blood glucose during infusion of fructose. If insulin is lacking about half of a fructose infusion can be converted to lactate and so contribute to a metabolic acidosis. This hazard is greatest in infants.

Changes in electrolyte balances must be anticipated during carbohydrate infusion. Beal et al (1953) reported that three times as much sodium and almost twice as much potassium was lost in the urine with fructose than with comparable glucose solutions. When fructose is infused pyruvate levels have been found to rise more rapidly than with glucose. This is an index of rapid utilisation and phosphorization and accounts for the rapid anti-ketogenic action of fructose. Glucose and fructose must remain the main contributors to calories from carbohydrate sources.

Sorbitol or glucitol is a sugar alcohol which is converted to fructose during body metabolism. Sorbitol is available in 10 and 20% solutions.

The pH is high and it is moderately irritant to vein walls. It is poorly absorbed by the renal tubules and thus has osmotic diuretic properties. Due to the addition of two extra carbon atoms in the sorbitol molecule its calorie yield is about 8 % greater than glucose or fructose. Sorbitol is a useful source of calories and large numbers can be given easily in moderate volumes. But its superiority over glucose has yet to be determined.

A pentose sugar xylotol, which is an intermediate in carbohydrate metabolism, has been used as a calorie source in parenteral nutrition. Xylotol is metabolised mainly in the liver and does not cause any change in blood glucose or insulin. The pentose phosphate cycle utilising xylotol is separate from the normal pathways of glucose metabolism and is linked to it at one point only. There is good evidence for the utilisation of this sugar by the body but toxicity has been reported following its use (Meng and Law, 1971).

Each of the alternative sources of carbohydrate, fructose, sorbitol and xylotol, have theoretical advantages over glucose and in a few situations may be useful but it is hard to find good reasons for passing over glucose as the main source of calories in any programme of parenteral feeding.

Indications for Parenteral Feeding

Patients who cannot use the alimentary canal for long periods of time or who have permanent intestinal damage due to conditions like Crohn's disease or have had massive intestinal resections can be considered as suffering from chronic alimentary failure. These patients will eventually die if they do not receive nutritional support by the parenteral route. Patients who for short periods of time after major injury or operation cannot take their requirements by mouth can be considered as an example of acute alimentary insufficiency (Johnston 1970, Allen and Lee, 1969).

Intestinal Indications

Severe extra renal losses of nitrogen occur in ulcerative colitis and Crohn's disease. Faecal losses of 10 or more grams per day can occur in the acute phase of ulcerative colitis and about half of the total body excretion of nitrogen can occur in the faeces in patients with Crohn's disease. Keeping pace with these alimentary losses can be difficult, many patients are toxic and anorexic and forced oral feeding only aggravates their intestinal problems. Full parenteral nutrition can be of considerable benefit pending either the onset of a further remission or the staging of a planned surgical procedure. Weight gains occur when adequate calories are given, serum albumin levels rise and the cumulative positive nitrogen balance which can be achieved in the absence of oedema is indicative of a significant increase in lean body mass (Fig. 43). A 2–8 fold increase of albumin synthesis rate has been observed after intravenous administration of amino acids in mal-nourished patients with low serum albumin levels.

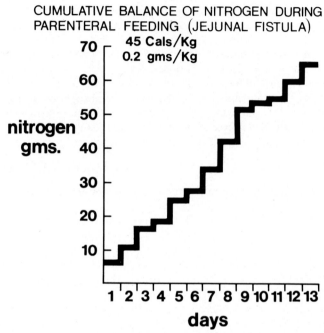

FIG. 43. Cumulative nitrogen balance during parenteral feeding.

Schuberth and Wretlind (1961) maintained the nutrition of a young man with Crohn's disease for five months by parenteral means during which time 10 kg of Soya bean oil emulsion was infused intravenously without any side effects. Dudrick et al (1968) has shown that intravenous nutrients can produce normal weight and growth patterns in babies with alimentary failure. Patients who are underweight at the time of surgery can benefit by the maintenance of an adequate intravenous intake of nutrients in the postoperative period. A positive balance of nitrogen is achieved easily in undernourished patients who show only a very small catabolic response to operation (Fig. 13).

Fistulae

The management of enterocutaneous fistulae of the small intestine is simplified by parenteral nutritional support. The losses from fistulae are reduced when oral intake is stopped and the nutritional state can be improved over a period of 6–8 weeks during which healing may occur if no distal obstruction is present and any intra-abdominal abscesses can be located and drained. Subsequent surgical closure will be required in some patients and successful operations have been reported with swift recovery after 4 or 5 weeks of complete parenteral nutrition.

Electrolyte balance and plasma protein levels require to be measured frequently during parenteral feeding in patients with large alimentary losses. As well as potassium, magnesium may be lost. Magnesium is an intracellular cation essential for the initiation of wound healing and when it is absent protein synthesis is poor.

Some patients with alimentary failure can provide some of their requirements by the oral route; and in these parenteral support assumes an adjuvant role. About half the requirements may be given orally and the rest intravenously. Excessive use of the oral route often causes excessive fluid losses from fistula and dehydration may develop.

Renal Failure

The need for supplies of intravenous calories in the management of renal failure is well recognised (Blagg, 1967).

The management of acute renal failure is complicated often by malnutrition. Anorexia, repeated trauma and sespis all contribute to the nutritional deficit. Biochemical equilibrium can often be maintained by repeated dialysis but survival can be threatened by the inability to control nutrition while waiting for recovery of renal function. The addition of amino acids to the extent of 40 grams of protein and over 2,000 calories daily reduces the catabolic rate but does not cause an increase in the rate of rise of blood urea. Intravenous fat can be given during renal failure but not immediately before haemodialysis because the dialysing membrane becomes covered by a thin layer of fat emulsion which prevents any exchange taking place. The view that infusions of fat emulsions might interfere with cellular recovery in the kidney has not been confirmed. No alterations in renal plasma flow or free water clearance has been observed following parenteral feeding.

Neck Surgery

There are some situations where in spite of normal alimentary canal parenteral nutrients can be of great benefit. Patients having major surgery for the treatment of malignant disease of the mouth, pharynx and larynx cannot always be maintained by nasogastric tube feeding and gastrostomy is not always desirable. Postoperative intravenous feeding for the first week after such operations is essential.

Burns

Patients with burns lose large amounts of protein. After the acute phase when plasma proteins require rapid replacement a period of more gradual loss occurs when as much as 2 to 4 grams of protein/kg body weight will be required to maintain a positive balance of nitrogen. The alimentary route must be used initially to supply these needs but frequently large intakes are impossible, as diarrhoea develops when large volumes of hypertonic nutrients are given. The combined use of oral and intravenous feeding is then indicated in an attempt to maintain nutritional homeostasis.

Postoperative Complications

Patients who develop complications after major surgery often qualify for parenteral support. If in the first few days after operation it becomes clear that an adequate intake will not be possible for many days, then parenteral nutrients should be given. The most satisfactory way of determining the effectiveness of such support is to observe the maintenance of body weight. Nutritional support in undernourished patients requiring major surgery should commence 5 days before surgery and should be continued throughout the period of operation. Fat should probably not be used in the immediate postoperative period.

Paediatrics

The neonate can withstand short periods of deprivation of water and nutrients. The oral route usually becomes available but this is not possible as in prolonged ileus, massive resection for atresia and gastroschisis. Meticulous care is required in neonatal parenteral nutrition. Rickham (1967) and Dudrick et al (1968) indicate that growth can be produced by the use of parenteral nutrients in infants with alimentary insufficiency.

The role of parenteral nutrition in keeping up with the intestinal malabsorption of Crohn's disease and the exudative protein loss of ulcerative colitis is discussed on p. 192.

Designing an Intravenous Diet

When intravenous feeding is required decisions have to be taken regarding the choice of nutrient solution and the total requirements of calories, amino acids and carbohydrates.

Calorie requirements depend upon body weight activity and in surgical patients the presence of complications. Patients at rest in hospital require about 30–40 calories per kg per day. The normal daily intake of protein is around 60–70 g per day or about 1·0 g per kg per day and each gram of protein provides 4 calories. Protein should provide 10 to 15% of the calorie expenditure. The calorie contribution of infused amino acids is uncertain as they are not an immediate source of calories. Carbohydrate which yields 4 calories per gram during utilization accounts for 50% of the calorie requirements. The daily intake should be about 150 g (2 g per kg) which is half the amount of carbohydrate normally present in the body as glycogen.

The daily requirements depend initially upon body weight and suggested daily minimal needs for each kg of body weight in resting and catabolic situations are: shown in Table 20.

The daily fluid and electrolyte balance must be calculated first and the nutritional balance adjusted to these needs.

The composition of currently available solutions are shown in Table 34. It must be remembered that while it is easy to give all the calories required in the form of fat emulsions, a proportion must be given as carbohydrate for purposes of protein incorporation. Some intravenous fat solutions contain glycerol and others sorbitol. These substances are metabolised in the carbohydrate pathways. The need for the simultaneous infusion of amino acids and carbohydrates has been stressed and because of this amino acid solutions containing carbohydrate calories are available. The optimum calorie to nitrogen ratio for the maintenance of nitrogen balance appears to be about 200 calories per g of nitrogen infused. It is sometimes necessary to add electrolytes to parenteral nutrients. This practice is not without the risk of introducing infection and additions must only be made to amino acid or carbohydrate solutions and not to fat in order to prevent the break up of the emulsion and the production of fat emboli. The pH of some of the solutions used is low but Peaston (1967) has found no alteration in the acid base balance during parenteral feeding and the rapid breakdown of parenteral fat has not been found to significantly raise blood ketone levels. Nevertheless in acutely ill patients with either a metabolic or respiratory acidosis the infusion of law pH solutions might create acid base problems. The sodium concentration of the casein hydrolysates is high and must be remembered in post operative patients. The electrolyte concentrations of the synthetic mixtures is more appropriate for ill patients.

Technique of Administration

The technique of infusion is of considerable importance. Thrombophlebitis can occur in about 80% of patients when peripheral veins are used for several days for the infusion of amino acid solutions and carbohydrate solutions are even more damaging. Fat emulsions do not appear to have any irritant action on veins. The addition of heparin and hydrocortisone to the solutions has been suggested but it is difficult to find any evidence of the advantages of these additions.

If parenteral nutrition is to be maintained for more than a few days, then an indwelling catheter should be placed in a large vein under strict aseptic conditions to avoid the frequent changes of peripheral

Table 34.
Composition of Some Parenteral Nutrients in Current Use

Solution	Volume ml	Calories	Alcohol G	Fructose G	Glucose G	Sorbitol G	Soya-bean oil G	Cotton-seed oil G	Glycerol G	Amino acids G	Nitrogen G	Sodium mEq/litre	Potassium mEq/litre	pH
Intralipid 10%	1000	1100					100		25					7
Intralipid 20%	1000	2000					200		25					7
Lipiphysan 10%	1000	1240				50		100						
Lipiphysan 15%	1000	1780				50		150						
Aminosol 10%	1000	320								100	12.7	160	0.5	5.6
Aminosol Fructose Ethanol	1000	875	25	150						33	4.2	54	0.1	5.6
Vamin 7%	1000	650		100						70	9.4	50	20	5.2
Trophysan 10	1000	534				99				40	6.7	6	8	6.4
Glucose 5%	1000	200			50									4.0
Fructose 20%	1000	800		200										4.0
Sorbitol 30%	1000	1200				300								7.0

infusion sites. Infusions can be maintained for a number of weeks by this means.

Septicaemia is a common problem after several weeks of intravenous feeding. Infection arises either from contamination of bottles of nutrients when electrolytes are being added, or by the entry of organisms at the junction between the skin and catheter. Blood cultures are often positive and organisms are often to be found in the fibrin clot around the tip of the catheter. This complication can be prevented by the use of a millipore filter in the infusion line and by the maintenance of a continuous antiseptic barrier at the point of entry of the catheter. Dudrick et al (1968) has kept patients free of infection for many months by means of filters. Infusions should be discontinued when fever develops and the intravenous catheter withdrawn.

The Artificial Gut

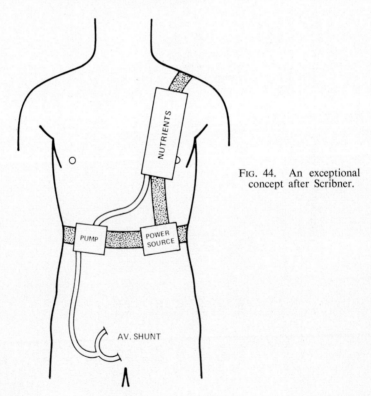

FIG. 44.   An exceptional concept after Scribner.

Where very prolonged intravenous nutrition is contemplated and vein thrombosis seems likely, then it may be necessary to insert an arteriovenous shunt in either the arm or leg or in some patients to surgically produce an arteriovenous fistula as an entry point into the circulation.

The long term use of intravenous feeding could be made simpler by the development of a system which can be strapped to the body. Scribner has developed a system for portable use in which a pump power unit and a supply of nutrients are fixed to a harness which is worn by the patient, the nutrient line being connected to an arterio-venous shunt (Fig. 44). The dilution of the nutrients in the fast flowing shunts will allow high concentrations of substances such as glucose to be used and 50% glucose solutions have been given for many days with success by this means. Problems which face the long term use of this artificial gut include infection and clotting. However, the develop-ment of this concept will enable patients to be maintained for months at a time in good nutritional condition while surgical procedures are carried out to restore normal alimentary function.

Side Effects

The side effects of parenteral nutrients may either be acute or develop late and insidiously (Table 36). Anaemia can develop during prolonged infusions of fat emulsions. The aetiology of the anaemia is uncertain but it is probably haemolytic but decreased erythropoiesis has also been reported during fat infusions.

Table 36.
Side Effects of Parenteral Nutrition

ACUTE EFFECTS	
COLLOID REACTION	Back and chest pain dyspnoea
PYROGENIC REACTION	Shivering and fever
CIRCULATORY EFFECTS	Flushing
MISCELLANEOUS	Nausea, vomiting, headache
LATE EFFECTS	
Prolonged coagulation time	Bleeding tendency Anaemia
I.V. Fat pigment	Liver dysfunction

Bleeding tendencies are well recognised in animal studies with fat infusions and have been reported clinically. Meng and Kaley (1965) observed a prolongation of the clotting time in some patients during parenteral feeding. Clot retraction can be reduced but fibrinogen levels have been unaffected. Thrombocytopenia has also been observed during fat infusions.

Other authors (Amris et al, 1964 and Lawson, 1965) have on the other hand drawn attention to increased coagulability of blood during fat infusions which appeared to be related to an increased rate of production of thrombin. Heparin has been given by some to obviate this problem. Reid and Ingram (1967) found little evidence of thrombus formation with fat emulsions. The disorders of coagulation and anaemia appear to be relatively minor and capable of correction.

Fat emulsions are a potential hazard to liver function during prolonged use in ill patients. The serum alkaline phosphatase will rise, the B.S.P. retention will increase and jaundice may develop. Liver biopsies after some weeks show intravenous brown fat pigment in the Küpfer cells. Similar pigment can be found in the spleen. The pigment is insoluble in most fat solvents and its significance is unknown.

Acute reactions during infusions of both fats and amino acids have been reported. The incidence of acute toxicity in less than 3% of infusions and includes a combination of symptoms:— pain in the back and chest, dyspnoea, headache, tachycardia, flushing, pyrexia, nausea and vomiting have all been reported. The symptoms cease when the infusion is discontinued. Fat is frequently given in association with other solutions and it is difficult in many reports to assess how much the infusion of other substances such as amino acids has been responsible for the symptoms. The frequency of these acute reactions is very low and of minor importance with the present fat emulsions.

Hypertonic solutions of carbohydrates and, in particular, Sorbitol have an osmotic diuretic action on the renal tubules and potassium may be lost in considerable amounts during infusion. A good review of all the problems of parenteral nutrition has been provided by Meng and Law (1970).

Laboratory Difficulties

Intravenous fats and amino acids can affect the accuracy of a number of biochemical investigations. Haemoglobin estimations during fat infusions are inaccurate as hyperlipaemia will interfere with colorimetric methods. Peptides in casein hydrolysates will interfere with the biuret reaction for measuring total plasma proteins and give an abnormally high result. Amino acids can also interfere with the diazo reaction for bilirubin and lead to high readings. Flame photometry on hyperlipaemic blood can be difficult and autoanalysers can also be blocked. If it is not possible to withhold intravenous amino acids and fats for 4 hours before taking a blood sample, then fat should be cleared from the plasma by dissolving it in ether.

Intestinal Tube Feeding

It is always desirable to use the alimentary canal for nutritional purposes whenever possible. The intake of all surgical patients can be increased by the use of concentrated, flavoured glucose solutions such as Hycal which contains between 2 and 3 calories per ml, milk with

Table 37.
2,000-Calorie Feed for Maintenance Purposes

Ingredient	Quantity	Protein (g)	Fat (g)	Carbohydrate (g)	Calories
Cow's milk	2,000 ml	68	74	96	1,320
50% fat emulsion	100 ml	—	50	—	465
Lactose	60 g	—	—	63*	236
Water	400 ml	—	—	—	—
Total		68	124	159	2,021

Weight of feed = 2,617 g   Volume of feed 2,500 ml   Water content = 2,400 ml (approx.)
Sodium content = 50 mEq   Potassium content = 80 mEq   *Calculate as monosaccharide.

3,000-Calorie Feed for Full Nourishment

Ingredient	Quantity	Protein (g)	Fat (g)	Carbohydrate (g)	Calories
Cow's milk	1,000 ml	34	37	48	660
50% fat emulsion	270 ml	—	135	—	1,236
Lactose	250 g	—	—	262*	983
Milk protein	35 g	35	—	—	144
Water	1,700 ml	—	—	—	—
Total		69	172	310	3,023

Weight of feed = 3,273 g   Volume of feed = 2,970 ml   Water content = 2,800 ml (approx.)
Sodium content 2 = 5 mEq   Potassium content = 40 mEq   To increase protein intake to 100 g day add
130 g milk protein. To increase protein intake to 300 g day add 230 g milk protein.   *Calculated as monosaccharide.

added carbohydrate and protein preparations such as Complan. These high calorie foods are often unpalatable to the very ill and nasogastric intubation may be required for nutritional support particularly in unconscious or unco-operative patients.

A maintenance diet with an intake of 0·16 g nitrogen and 30–40 calories per kg per day can be given into a gastrostomy tube without complications. When the nitrogen content is increased to 0·3 g/kg and the calories to 50 per kg per day diarrhoea occurs. Diarrhoea is a major problem when a jejunostomy is being used for feeding because the osmolar equilibrating mechanisms of stomach and duodenum have been bypassed. The osmolality of a tube feed should be kept as close as possible to 300 m Osm per litre. Carbohydrates, particularly lactose and electrolytes, have the greatest effect on osmolality. High protein feeds require extra calories and a calorie nitrogen ratio of 200:1 must be maintained if adequate utilisation is to be achieved even in nutritionally depleted patients.

Milk which is almost isotonic with plasma is an ideal component of a tube feed particularly if the feeding tube is situated in the jejunum. Milk is deficient in sugar and the addition of carbohydrate and electrolytes to the feed increases the osmotic pressure of the feed and increases the risk of diarrhoea. Lactose is the carbohydrate of choice; it has a higher molecular weight than sucrose or glucose and therefore weight for weight it will exert a lower osmotic pressure. However, the presence of alactasia in the intestinal cells of some debilitated patients must not be forgotten. Lactose is used widely, up to 250 g can be tolerated daily in a tube feed by most adults. The daily sodium content should be about 25 mEq and potassium around 50 mEq for most situations (Masterton et al, 1963).

Palatability is an important consideration; first, to avoid an unpleasant regurgitant taste in the mouth in patients fed by tube; secondly, to allow the same formula to be used for oral supplements or a total oral feed in those who can take liquids. For the latter reason it is wise to base the feed on fresh, powdered, or tinned milk, which most people can tolerate, if not enjoy. Crude protein preparations should be avoided and a fine suspension—for example, "Casilan"—should be used. Lactose is a satisfactory carbohydrate because it is not intolerably sweet. A small-particle fat emulsion ("prosparol") is virtually tasteless and suitable for addition to any tube feed, Table 37.

Medium chain triglycerides are broken down in the intestine more rapidly than normal fats, bile and pancreatic lipase are not absolutely essential for the hydrolysis of these substances (Holt, 1967). Medium chain triglycerides are carried in the portal vein after absorption. These compounds are now being added to mixtures of milk protein, egg albumin and sugar to provide a balanced easily absorbed liquid diet (Triosorbin).

REFERENCES

Beal, J. M., Smith, J. L. and Frost, P. M. (1953). Studies in the utilisation of fructose administered intravenously in man. *Surgery* **33**, 721.

Johnston, I. D. A. (1971). Parenteral Feeding. *Practitioner*, **206**, 103.

Allen, P. C. and Lee, H. A. (1969). A clinical guide to intravenous nutrition. Blackwell. London & Edinburgh.

Schuberth, O. and Wretlind, K. A. J. (1961). Intravenous infusions of fat emulsions, phosphatides and emulsifying agents. *Acta chir. scand. Suppl.* **278**, 3.

Dudrick, S. J., Welmore, D. W., Vars, H. M. and Rhoads, J. E. (1968). Long term total parenteral nutrition with growth development and positive nitrogen balance. *Surgery*, **64**, 134.

Blagg, C. R. (1967). The management of acute intrinsic reversible renal failure. *Postgrad. med. J.* **43**, 189.

Rickham, P. P. (1967). Massive small bowel resection in newborn infants. *Ann. roy. Coll. Surg. Engl.* **41**, 6, 480.

Peaston, M. J. T. (1967). Maintenance of metabolism during intensive patient care. *Postgrad. med. J.* **43**, 217.

Meng, H. G. and Kaley, J. S. (1965). Effect of multiple infusion of fat emulsion on blood coagulation. *Amer. J. clin. Nutr.* **16**, 157.

Amris, C. J., Brøckner, J. and Larsen, V. (1964). Changes in the coagulability of blood during infusion of intralipid. *Acta chir. scand. Suppl.* **325**, 70.

Hodder, E. (1873). Transfusion of milk in cholera. *Practitioner* **10**, 14.

Henriques, V. and Andersen, W. (1913). Total parenteral nutrition by intravenous injection. *Z. Physiol. Chem.* **42**, 357.

Elman, R. (1939). Time factor in retention of nitrogen after intravenous injection of a mixture of amino acids. *Proc. Soc. exp. Biol.* **40**, 484.

Munro, H. N. (1963). Factors affecting requirements for carbohydrates, fat and amino acids. *Nutritio Dieta* **5**, 298.

Tweedle, D. E. F. and Johnston, I. D. A. (1971). A comparison of intravenous synthetic amino acids and casein hydrolysates in postoperative patients. *Brit. J. Surg.* In press.

Wretlind, K. A. J. (1957). Effect of tributyrin on respiration and circulation. *Acta physiol. Scand.* **40**, 59.

Edgren, B. and Wretlind K. A. J. (1963). The theoretical background of the intravenous nutrition with fat emulsion. *Nutritio et dieta* **5**, 364.

Halberg, D., Schuberth, O. and Wretlind, K. A. J. (1966). Experimental and clinical studies with fat emulsions for intravenous nutrition. *Nutritio et dieta* **8**, 3, 245.

Lawson, L. J. (1965). Parenteral nutrition in surgery. *Brit. J. Surg.* **52**, 795.

Reid, D. J. and Ingram, G. I-C. (1967). Changes in blood coagulation during infusion of intralipid. *Clin. Sci.* **33**, 399.

Holt, P. R. (1967). Medium chain triglycerides—A useful adjunct in nutritional therapy. *Gastroenterology* **53**, 961.

Masterton, J. P., Dudley, H. A. F. and MacRae, S. (1963). Alimentary tube feeding. *Brit. med. J.* **2**, 909.

Meng, H. C. and Law, D. H. (1971). Parenteral nutrition. (Proceedings of an International Symposium.) Charles C. Thomas, Springfield, Illinois.

14: Endocrine Problems

The endocrine system is of surgical importance because the syndromes associated with excessive production of hormones by hyperplastic or tumorous glands are often treated by surgical removal, and endocrine hypofunction or insufficiency can jeopardise survival of postoperative patients (Chapter 4).

The diagnosis and surgical management of endocrine disorders are outside the scope of this book but some of the common metabolic disorders associated with the endocrine glands will be discussed.

Pituitary Ablation

The pituitary gland is often removed surgically for primary disease or ablated by irradiation in patients with metastatic breast carcinoma. Atrophy of all the target glands follows removal but health can be maintained by appropriate substitution therapy.

Cortisone acetate is given before and immediately after operation by injection. Pure glucocorticoids such as prednisone is inadequate replacement in some patients and the addition of the electrocorticoid 5 α fluhydrocortisone is required. Thyroid deficiency develops slowly and 0·2–0·3 μg of thyroxine daily will be required after a few weeks.

Polyuria frequently begins immediately after operation and sometimes stops spontaneously after a few days indicating that complete destruction of the post-pituitary has not occurred. When polyuria and polydipsia persist pitressin tannate has to be given either in the form of tannate and oil, or as snuff. Diabetes insipidus often disappears after several months and it is unusual for it to be a permanent problem. This remission of symptoms is due to that fact that the supra-optic nucleus secretes the hormone. The neurohypophysis is a functioning entity consisting of the hypothalama-neurohypophyseal system, only part of which is destroyed at hypophysectomy.

Adrenocortical Overactivity

Cushing's syndrome is due to excess cortisol in the circulation. Some patients will also exhibit signs of excess androgens in the blood.

Bilateral adrenal hyperplasia is the commonest cause of the syndrome. The clinical features consist of hypertension, obesity, change of facial appearance, hyperglycaemia, muscle weakness, osteoporosis and menstrual irregularity. The diagnosis is simple in some and difficult in others (Welbourn et al, 1971). The most reliable method of establishing the diagnosis of Cushing's syndrome is to measure the cortisol production rate by means of an isotope dilution technique. The absence of diurnal rhythm in the plasma cortisol levels and high outputs of 17 hydroxycorticosteroids in the urine are found in Cushing's syndrome.

When over production of cortisol has been established, the origin of the causative lesion must be sought. Bilateral adrenal hyperplasia can be treated at the pituitary or adrenal level. Patients who have had adrenalectomy require permanent replacement therapy with cortisol and a mineralocorticoid. About 10% will develop pigmentation of the skin and enlargement of the pituitary fossa usually due to a chromophobe adenoma. Patients on maintenance steroids must be warned about the nature of their treatment and the necessity of maintaining treatment at all times.

Adrenocortical Insufficiency

Adrenal failure results when insufficient amounts of cortisol and aldosterone are available for the needs of the body. Failure may be either acute as after adrenalectomy or chronic as in Addison's disease. Adequate amounts of adrenocortical hormones are required for normal recovery after injury otherwise peripheral circulatory failure will develop and death may follow if the condition is unrecognised and is not treated. The failure of the adrenal cortex to respond to injury in a normal manner may be either primary and confined to the adrenal or secondary when the primary problem is in the pituitary.

Primary Adrenal Failure

Addison's Disease

The recognition of Addison's disease in surgical patients is most important as otherwise minor injuries or surgical procedures may be followed by acute circulatory collapse. The presence of low blood pressure, hyponatraemia, patchy brown pigmentation and loss of body hair are important signs.

Adrenal Infarction

Severe trauma to the chest and posterior abdominal wall sometimes causes haemorrhage to occur into the adrenal with destruction and loss of function. Similar haemorrhagic destruction occurs in the newborn after birth trauma and in infants with meningococcal septicaemia. The technique of retrograde venography of the adrenals used to search for small cortical tumours can be complicated by haemorrhagic destruction of the glands.

Cross clamping of the aorta above the level of the adrenals during the resection of a difficult aortic aneurysm may infarct both adrenals.

Virilising Hyperplasia

Patients with this rare condition have a relative deficiency of cortisol due to a block in normal synthesis. The deficiency may only be detected during the demands of a surgical operation. When virilisation is due to a cortical adenoma, insufficiency is unlikely as the remaining adrenal functions normally.

"Exhaustion"

It was considered that patients after very severe injuries with prolonged recovery or with numerous complications after surgery were liable to develop adrenal exhaustion with severe hypotension, particularly if further sudden demands were made on the adrenal cortex. Many patients in these situations respond to intravenous injections of cortisol with restoration of the blood pressure to normal. Cope (1964) reviewed this problem of adrenal insufficiency or exhaustion and felt that the condition was uncommon and that the majority of patients who succumbed died from other causes. The adrenal cortex normally responds to prolonged stress by hypertrophy. Sampson and Brooke (1963) measured the plasma cortisol levels in such patients and invariably found them to be raised. The diagnosis of adrenal exhaustion can only be made when low levels of plasma cortisol are found. McInnes et al (1971) demonstrated that unexpectedly low plasma cortisol levels were found in a minority of very ill people. Low levels in these patients were found to be unresponsive to ACTH stimulations. Adrenal insufficiency thus proven responds to a cortisol infusion.

Secondary Adrenal Failure

Secondary adrenal or primary pituitary failure is due to hypopituitarism or hypophysectomy, and inhibition by therapy with corticosteroids or ACTH. Secondary adrenal failure is less rapid in onset than the primary type, because the production of aldosterone is relatively unaffected.

Patients who have had treatment with steroids are liable to develop insufficiency. Failure has been reported more than one year after withdrawal of treatment but it barely seems justifiable to give steroid cover during and after operation to all patients and a pre-operative test to detect those who will require steroids at the time of surgery is indicated. The adrenal may be stimulated by injection of ACTH with measurements of the changes in plasma cortisol levels. This test however only demonstrates adrenal capacity and gives no information about the ability of the pituitary adrenal axis to respond to stress. Carter and James (1970) have shown that a positive response to insulin hypoglycaemia as measured by a rise in the plasma cortisol level is a valuable index in at risk patients of the capacity of their hypothalamic pituitary adrenal axis to respond to the stress of surgery.

Patients with established adrenal insufficiency from whatever cause or those undergoing total adrenalectomy require careful regulation of steroid dosage during and after surgery:— day before operation— 100 mg cortisone acetate I.M.; day of operation—100 mg cortisone acetate I.M. and 100 mg hydrocortisone hemisuccinate just before surgery. This dose should be repeated in four hours in major procedures and in patients on high pre-operative maintenance doses of steroids. Any unexplained fall in the blood pressure in the first twenty-four hours should be treated at once by 100 mg hydrocortisone I.V., on the day after operation—100 mg cortisone acetate should be given intramuscularly. As soon as oral feeding has been resumed 25 mg cortisone by mouth twice daily should be sufficient until the pre-operative programme is re-established.

Factors other than an increase in circulating cortisol maintain the blood pressure after injury because many patients who had had glucocorticoids failed to show any increase in circulating cortisol levels in the plasma after operation without developing any fall in blood pressure.

Acute adrenal insufficiency should only be diagnosed when hypovolaemia has been excluded. 100 mg hydrocortisone should be given intravenously after removing a blood sample for cortisol estimation, which can now be measured quickly. Hydrocortisone can then be added to intravenous fluids and 100 mg given immediately and continued at a rate of 100 mg six hourly.

The absence of a response makes the diagnosis of adrenal insufficiency unlikely.

Parathyroid

Hypocalcaemia with tingling of extremities and tetany may follow surgery on the parathyroids and thyroid. Hypokalaemia and hypomagnesaemia may also be associated with hypocalcaemia. The level of serum calcium at which symptoms and signs are present varies greatly. Patients with renal failure failure who are acidotic can tolerate very low levels of calcium such as 5 mg/100 ml or less with little or no discomfort.

The development of tingling with a positive Chvostek or Trousseau's sign in patients following neck surgery is an indication for the slow I.V. injection of 10–20 ml of 10% solution of calcium gluconate. These injections may have to be repeated at intervals. Supplementary oral calcium should be given. Calcium Sandoz (calcium gluconogalactogluconate) is a useful preparation. The tablets are effervescent and each contains 380 mg of calcium.

Vitamin D may also be required but it is advisable to commence with small doses such as 20,000 I.U. daily, increasing to 50,000 to 100,000 units in some patients depending on the level of the serum calcium. A.T. 10 (dihydro tachysterol) in doses of 0·5–2·0 mg/day may be used as an alternative and has some attractions as its activity more closely resembles parathormone. If vitamin D or A.T. 10 therapy is excessive and hypercalcaemia occurs renal damage may ensue. Such hypercalcaemia will respond to cortisone by injection. The serum magnesium levels should be checked during treatment of hypocalcaemia as they are sometimes low and supplemental magnesium will be necessary.

Pancreas

Diabetic patients can undergo either emergency or elective surgical operations provided their insulin requirements are controlled carefully.

Elective Surgery

Patients on diet alone should have blood sugar levels checked at frequent intervals after surgery. Insulin may be needed if control is unsatisfactory. Patients on oral hypoglycaemic agents should be given soluble insulin before operation and return to oral drugs as soon as possible after surgery.

Patients requiring insulin should be stabilised before and after surgery on soluble insulin. The operation should commence as soon as possible after the morning dose of insulin and an intravenous infusion of 5% glucose given throughout the operation and for as long as it is required afterwards.

Insulinomas or β cell tumours of the pancreas cause severe hypoglycaemia. The medical management of hypoglycaemia consists of giving insulin antagonists like A.C.T.H., cortisone or growth hormone. A long acting preparation of glucagon has also been used with success. An oral drug diazoxide has also been found valuable in controlling intractible hypoglycaemia in patients with malignant insulinomas. The effectiveness of this drug in controlling hypoglycaemia should be assessed before surgery in case no tumour can be identified.

Patients undergoing exploration of insulinomas should have an intravenous infusion of glucose running throughout to prevent dangerous hypoglycaemia developing under anaesthesia. Blood glucose should be monitored throughout. As it rises significantly within 10–15 minutes of the complete removal of an insulinoma.

It is thus possible to confirm biochemically that all functioning tumour tissue has been removed. The blood glucose continues to climb for several days after the successful removal of an insulinoma and insulin may be required to control ketosis. The necessity to resect the body and tail of the pancreas as a blind procedure has gone. The results of distal blind resection are poor as many tumours lie hidden in the head as in the tail and a blind resection is often the prelude to total pancreatectomy if the lesion is located in the head on a later occasion.

Adrenal Medulla

Phaeochromocytoma although present in less than 1 % of the hypertensive population must frequently be in the surgeon's mind. The symptoms are variable depending on the proportion of adrenaline and noradrenaline in the secretions and the diagnosis can be elusive. Sustained hypertension is the commonest presenting feature. The fasting blood glucose is often high and the glucose tolerance test abnormal. Paroxysmal hypertension is less common and when present is accompanied by attacks of headaches, weakness, sweating, nervousness and tremor. On occasions the metabolic effects of adrenaline take precedence over the vascular effects and the clinical picture may resemble thyrotoxicosis. A number of deaths have been reported in patients with unsuspected phaeochromocytomas undergoing elective operations for other conditions. These patients often have diminished circulatory volume due to persistent action of noradrenaline on the peripheral vascular bed and they withstand blood loss badly. The induction of anaesthesia sometimes is enough to precipitate a hypertensive crisis. If such an event should occur during surgery, the operation should be abandoned forthwith and volume expanders given until blood pressure has been restored.

Patients undergoing exploration for phaeochromocytoma require careful preparation. The α blocking agent phenoxybenzamine is given intravenously for 2 or 3 days before operation. The use of this substance often leads to a significant increase in the circulating plasma volume. β blocking agents such as propranolol have been found effective in controlling cardiac arrhythmias in some. The maintenance of blood volume is an important objective during surgery. Transfusion should commence early in the procedure and any fall in blood pressure treated by an increase in the rate of transfusion. Adrenaline and noradrenaline should not be given to counteract hypotension in the postoperative period. Some neuroblastomas in infants have been shown to excrete pressor amines and hypotensive crises can occur during removal. The metabolites of adrenaline and noradrenaline should be measured in the urine of children with this tumour and appropriate blocking agents used if high levels are recorded.

Thyroid

It is important to assess the function of the thyroid clinically and biochemically before undertaking any surgery on the gland. It is also important to recognise under and overactivity in patients with surgical problems unrelated to the thyroid.

Tests of thyroid function consist of measuring the trapping of iodide by the gland. The amount of radioiodine taken up by the gland depends on the level of iodine in the plasma and other sites in the body. The release of thyroid hormone from the gland can also be measured by means of radioiodine. The T_3 resin uptake test consists of the addition of labelled Triiodothyronine T_3 to samples of plasma. The number of free binding sites on the plasma proteins not occupied by thyroid hormone can be measured. This test is a useful measure of plasma thyroid hormone levels. Hall et al, 1969.

Thyroid Crises

Thyroid storm or crisis is no longer a problem in the surgical management of thyrotoxicosis but in a few patients with severe hyperthyroidism pre-operative control may be difficult and a risk of thyroid storm is present. The syndrome, well known in the early days of thyroid surgery, consists of high fever, tachycardia, severe restlessness and convulsions. Atrial fibrillation and heart failure may develop later. The release of very large amounts of thyroxine into the circulation leads to excessive oxidative phosphorylation and energy expenditure. This expenditure is uncontrollable and is manifested as heat gain to the body rather than useful work or the production of further energy stores. The effect is similar to malignant hyperpyrexia (p. 239). Treatment consists of large doses of iodide by mouth and 10 mg should be given four hourly. Sympathetic blocking drugs such as propranolol are valuable in reducing sympathetic overactivity.

Hypoparathyroidism may develop after operation due probably to interference with the blood supply of the parathyroids. The treatment of the associated tetany has been described (p. 233).

Hypothyroidism

Elderly patients with unrecognised myxoedema often have surgical problems. They are very accident prone and often turn up in the Accident Department. The recognition and treatment of the myxoedema will make any subsequent surgery much safer.

Depression is a common problem in many myxoedematous patients. Apart from mental sluggishness, weight gain, constipation, cold intolerance are other important points in the history. Rough dry skin with a yellowish tint and signs of peripheral circulatory insufficiency are useful signs. Too much reliance should not be placed on eyebrow thinning. Myxoedema is usually recognised when the patient is first observed or not at all.

The most valuable screening test for hypothyroidism is the protein bound iodine and a value of less than 3 μg/100 ml is good evidence of underactivity. The T_3 resin uptake is another useful test.

Endocrine Syndromes and Malignant Disease

Many different hormones can be secreted by malignant tumours and the associated endocrine syndromes present and often require urgent attention before the underlying malignancy is obvious. These syndromes are being recognised with increasing frequency.

Ectopic A.C.T.H. Syndrome

The ectopic A.C.T.H. syndrome is perhaps the most widely recognised and occurs usually in association with lung, thymic and pancreatic tumours mainly and the endocrine problem may be recognised before the underlying malignant disease produces any symptoms. The Cushing's syndrome may develop rapidly but the biochemical changes overshadow the clinical picture and hypokalaemic alkalosis is usually present due to a marked increase in secretion of cortisol. The plasma and urinary cortisol levels in these patients are higher than in any other patients with Cushing's syndrome and are not influenced by dexamethasone, A.C.T.H. or Metyrapone. The prognosis is very poor and it is seldom possible to control their Cushing's syndrome adequately. However, the bronchial adenoma or carcinoid which is essentially benign produces the same picture. It is important that every effort be made to diagnose such a lesion as the treatment consists of removal of the bronchial adenoma rather than adrenalectomy. Patients with gross overstimulation of the adrenal cortex can be helped by the anticonvulsant drug Aminoglutethimide in a dose of 1–1½ grams daily. This substance blocks the production of cortisol by the adrenal. The effect however may be only temporary.

Hypoglycaemia

Some patients with primary tumours of the liver or slow growing connective tissue tumours in the abdomen or mediastinum are associated with hypoglycaemia. The hypoglycaemia attacks are similar to those found with islet cell tumours of the pancreas. The syndrome appears to be due to the production of a hypoglycaemic agent by the tumour which is distinct from insulin. If the tumour is inoperable diazoxide may be of value.

Hypercalcaemia

Hypercalcaemia due to bone destruction is often unrecognised in patients with osseous metastases. However, hypercalcaemia can also occur in patients with malignant disease and no obvious bone disease (Carey, 1966). Treatment of some primary tumours led to the return of the serum calcium level to normal within a few days. These observations suggest that some humoral factor from the tumour was causing the hypercalcaemia and there is some evidence for the production of a substance with a parathormone like action (Sherwood et al, 1967). Severe hypercalcaemia in patients with malignant disease usually merits treatment and infusions of sodium phosphate, injections of corticosteroids and the use of chelating agents are often effective.

Inappropriate Antidiuretic Hormone

Dilutional hyponatremia is found occasionally in association with poorly differentiated lung cancers. This is due to the inappropriate production and secretion of antidiuretic hormone by the neoplasm (Bower et al, 1964). The serum sodium in this condition may fall to less than 120 mEq per litre. The haematocrit may be low and the blood urea may not be raised and the plasma volume may be increased. The patients will complain of drowsiness and mental confusion. These patients respond to restriction of water, the administration of an electrocorticoid (9 α fluorohydrocortisone) and sodium and potassium supplements.

Other less common endocrine syndromes associated with ectopic production of hormones include hyperthyroidism associated with trophoplastic tumours such as choriocarcinoma which may produce substances with T.S.H.-like activity. A number of patients have been reported with tumours secreting more than one hormone.

REFERENCES

Cope, C. L. (1964). Adrenal steroids and disease. London, Pitman Medical.

Carter, M. E. and James, V. H. T. (1970). Pituitary adrenal response to surgical stress in patients on A.C.T.H. *Lancet*, **1**, 328.

Sampson, P. A. and Brooke, B. N. (1963). Plasma cortisol levels in stress. *Lancet* **1**, 701.

McInnes, C., Rothwell, R. I., Jacobs, H. S. and Nabarro, J. D. N. (1971). *Lancet* 49.

Welbourn, R. B., Montgomery, D. A. D. and Kennedy, T. C. (1971). Natural History of Treated Cushing's Syndrome. *Brit. J. Surg.* **58**, 1.

Hall, R., Anderson, J. and Smart, G. A. (1969). Fundamentals of Clinical Endocrinology. London, Pitman medical.

Carey, V. C. (1966). Hypercalcaemia in Malignant Disease. *Amer. Rev. resp. Dis.* **93**, 584.

Sherwood, L. M., O'Riorden, J. L. H., Aurbach, G. D. and Potts,' J. T. (1967). Parathormone like substance in malignant disease. *J. clin. Endocrinol.* **27**, 140.

Bower, B. F., Mason, D. M. and Forsham, P. H. (1964). Inappropriate Secretion of Vasopressin. *New Eng. J. Med.*, **271**, 934.

15: Temperature Changes

Body temperature often fluctuates during anaesthesia and surgery, and is frequently raised in the postoperative period at a time when there is no evidence of infection (Roe, 1968).

General Anaesthesia

The heat regulating centre in the hypothalamus is paralysed temporarily during general anaesthesia and the patients are vulnerable to temperature changes. Some patients come to the operating theatre with a falling temperature following premedication. Factors which tend to lower body temperature during surgery are low ambient temperatures, of 16–21°C in operating areas and the exposure of internal organs for prolonged periods of time to a cool environment. Heat loss on the other hand is prevented by the surgical drapes which enclose an insulating envelope of air around the patient. Occasionally hyperpyrexia or heat stroke occurs if the temperature in operating rooms is very high especially during summer months. Predisposing factors for heat stroke during surgery are dehydration, a pre-existing fever and the use of closed circuit anaesthetic systems which recirculate warm moist gases through the patient's lungs. Hyperthermia under these conditions must be distinguished from the rare but highly lethal anaesthetic hyperthermia. This abnormal response occurs during anaesthesia with Halothane and muscle relaxants. Instead of paralysis of muscles generalised muscle rigidity occurs and a severe and rapid rise in body temperature follows. The syndrome can occur when relaxants have not been used and it is suggested that uncontrolled uncoupling of oxidation and phosphorylation with energy release is triggered off, by the anaesthetic agent resulting in greatly increased heat production. The syndrome has a mortality of about 60% and may occur sporadically or in families when an autosomal dominant pattern has been detected in connection with the defect. Raised levels of the enzyme creatine phosphokinase have been found in the serum of relatives of patients who have had malignant hyperpyrexia and screening may be possible in the future in selected groups to identify patients at risk (Denborough, 1970).

Postoperative Fever

It is not uncommon to find a modest rise in temperature in the first couple of days after operation without any evidence of infection.

It may be that the inflammatory response required to cope with blood clot and damaged tissue in the operation area is the cause of the modest changes in temperature but there is also evidence that when body temperature is monitored carefully and controlled during anaesthesia and surgery no postoperative fever occurs. This physiological fever or overswing following hypothermia during surgery and is of little clinical significance.

Fever after surgery is usually an indication of infection and the surgeon is more interested in temperature as a diagnostic index rather than the effects of the increased temperature alone. It is often the presenting sign of atelectasis and respiratory infection in the first few days after operation and may be due to the absorption of bacterial pyrogens from the occluded segments. Fever associated with massive collapse leads rapidly to other problems because the increased oxygen needs of the body due to raised temperature cannot be met due to respiratory insufficiency.

Infections in many closed spaces within the liver or in the subphrenic region are associated with spiking fever which may be due to the intermittent release of pyrogens into the blood stream.

Miscellaneous Causes

Compatible blood transfusion may be accompanied by an acute fever in about 3% of transfusions. The fever may be due to sensitivity to plasma (Mollison, 1956). A febrile reaction is characteristic of an incompatible transfusion. Pyrogens may be present on some occasions in the donor blood. Febrile reactions usually occur within the first hour of commencing a transfusion but sometimes within 5 to 10 minutes. Shivering and a feeling of cold may herald the pyrexia. After stopping the transfusion aspirin and antihistamines are useful in the control of the fever.

Dehydration is associated frequently with pyrexia. Fluid losses in some patients can be insidious and the fever is linked to diminished function of the heat loss mechanisms with, for example, a reduced capacity to sweat. Temperature will return to normal as fluid is given. This problem is more liable to develop in the very young or the elderly.

Fever can follow head injury and some neurosurgical procedures due probably to trauma and cerebral oedema in the hypothalamic pituitary area.

Metabolic Effects of Fever

The energy needs of the body are increased during fever and the extent of the increased demands depends upon the temperature changes. The metabolic rate is raised by about 13% for each 1°C increase in temperature and prolonged periods of pyrexia thus make considerable metabolic demands on the body.

The pulse rate usually follows the changes in body temperature during fever. This is a close relationship indicating that cardiac activity may be temperature sensitive. When the body temperature is low, severe peripheral constriction develops. There is also experimental evidence that the respiratory centre is very sensitive to temperature change.

The salicylates remain the most important drug for the reduction of body temperature. Phenothiazine derivatives such as chlorpromazine will lower the temperature due to its direct action on the hypothalamus and its inhibiting of thermoregulatory centres.

Hypothermia:— may be deliberate or accidental, as in preparation for surgery as occurs in elderly people living alone in poor accommodation.

Tolerance to circulatory arrest increases proportionally as cooling proceeds and induced hypothermia has facilitated much cardiac surgery.

The first reaction of the body to cold is to shiver to attempt to maintain the normal temperature. During anaesthesia of course shivering is abolished. The rate and depth of the respirations are reduced as the temperatures falls. Carbon dioxide is retained and progressive anoxia occurs. Organs with a rich blood supply such as the liver, brain and heart cool rapidly while muscle cools slowly. The heart slows as the temperature falls and arrhythmia and arrest will develop earlier in the elderly and much later in young children. The peripheral pulse becomes weak and may be imperceptible in profound hypothermia.

Cellular function in the liver and kidney is depressed and some substances such as lactate accumulate in the blood. During profound hypothermia to 10–15°C blood viscosity rises and sludging of blood cells occurs. The metabolic demand for oxygen falls and the oxygen content of venous blood rises.

Many factors continue to produce a metabolic acidosis during hypothermia. The acidosis may require correction with bicarbonate on rewarming. The plasma potassium level falls during cooling.

Controlled hypothermia allows up to 60 minutes of circulatory arrest for open heart surgery or neurosurgical procedure.

REFERENCES

Roe, C. F. (1968). Surgical aspects of Fever. Current problems in surgery. New Year Book.

Denborough, M. A. (1970). Creative phosphokinase levels in hyperpyrexia. *Lancet* **1,** 1138.

Mollison, P. C. (1956). Blood transfusion in clinical medicine. 2nd Edition. Oxford Blackwell **14,** 393.

Index

243